eClinical Trials

Planning & Implementation

Rebecca Daniels Kush, Ph.D.

and

Paul Bleicher, M.D., Ph.D.
Wayne R. Kubick
Stephen T. Kush
Ronald Marks, Ph.D.
Stephen A. Raymond, Ph.D.
Barbara Tardiff, M.D.

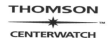

THOMSON

CENTERWATCH

22 Thomson Place · Boston, MA 02210
Phone (617) 856-5900 · Fax (617) 856-5901
www.centerwatch.com

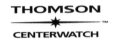

THOMSON
CENTERWATCH™

eClinical Trials: Planning & Implementation
by Rebecca Daniels Kush, Ph.D., and Paul Bleicher, M.D., Ph.D.,
Wayne R. Kubick, Stephen T. Kush, Ronald Marks, Ph.D.,
Stephen A. Raymond, Ph.D., Barbara Tardiff, M.D.

| **Editor** | **Publisher** | **Design** |
| Sara Gambrill | Ken Getz | Paul Gualdoni |

ISBN 1-930624-28-X

TABLE OF CONTENTS

Chapter 1   **Setting the Stage: An Overview** **9**
Clinical Trials—A Place to Begin 12

Chapter 2   **Today's Clinical Trial** **15**
Objectives 15
Introduction 15
The Clinical Research Cycle—Paper-Based 16
The Clinical Research Cycle—The Technology 23
    That Can Be Applied Today
Conclusion 35

Chapter 3   **The Optimal Electronic Clinical Trial—** **36**
A Vision for the Future
Objectives 36
Introduction 36
Goals for the Optimal Electronic Clinical Trial 37
The Vision—Putting It All Together 51
Conclusion 53

Chapter 4   **Process Redesign and Supporting Technologies** . .**54**
Objectives 54
Introduction 54
Shredding the Paper—Process Redesign 55
Metrics for Assessing Newly Introduced Technology . . .61
Supporting Technologies and Services for eCTs 63
Conclusion 69

Chapter 5   **Achieving eClinical Trials** **72**
Objectives 72
Introduction 72
Elements for Implementing eClinical Trials 73
Special Implementation Considerations for eCTs 78
Conclusion 79

Chapter 6   **Measuring and Managing for Success:** **80**
Metrics for Electronic Clinical Trials
Objectives 80
Introduction 80
Clinical Trials Metrics Collection 81
Conclusion 89

Chapter 7   **Performing Electronic Clinical Trials** **91**
in Accord with Regulations
Objectives 91
Agency Aim in Creating 21 CFR 11 92
Regulatory Considerations in Planning 94
   an Electronic Clinical Trial
Regulatory Considerations While Executing 100
   an Electronic Clinical Trial
Conclusion 106

Chapter 8   **Data Quality and Data Integrity** **108**
Objectives 108
Definitions of Data Quality and Data Integrity 109
Error Sources 109
Basic Principles 110
Conclusion 113

Chapter 9   **The Impact of eClinical Trial Technology** **114**
on Safety Surveillance and IRBs
Objectives 114
Time Delay 115
Responsibilities for Monitoring Patient Safety 115
Patient Privacy 121
Conclusion 123

Chapter 10 **Industry Data Standards: Ensuring the** **124**
Success of Electronic Clinical Trial
Implementations
Objectives 124
The Value of Standards 125
The CDISC Operational Data Model 130
Further Progress on Clinical Data Standards 132
Conclusion 132

Appendix A **Endnotes** **134**

Appendix B **Selected Reading** **137**

Appendix C **Glossary** **139**

Appendix D **Traceability Matrix** **156**

Appendix E **21 CFR Part 11** **163**

Appendix F **Guidance for Industry:** **171**
Computerized Systems Used
in Clinical Trials [CSUCT]

About CenterWatch **184**

About the Authors **191**

PLANNING

CHAPTER 1

Setting the Stage: An Overview

The rapid exchange of electronic information, the performance of electronic transactions and desire for access to real-time data are hallmarks of the new millennium. It is common today for most American and Western European households to have real-time access to financial and business data in order to make faster and more frequent decisions. On a daily basis, tens of millions of people perform business and personal electronic transactions—they make travel reservations on the web; they purchase automobiles, clothing and books; they manage their finances; and they buy and sell stocks. Many Americans will complete their federal income taxes online. We no longer have to go to a bank during working hours; we just use our ATM card at the automatic teller machine or connect from home to check our account status or pay bills. We consider it commonplace for a supplier to get approval to make a charge to our credit cards in a matter of seconds. The transaction data are immediately available for review. The area of finance—one of the most sensitive and confidential areas of our lives—has largely evolved to the point where the latest information technology is being used routinely to streamline the way transactions are conducted.

Contrast the way business is conducted in the financial industry with the way it is conducted in the healthcare industry. Most physicians do not have electronic access to patient records. In the case of a patient requiring emergency treatment outside of his or her health system, it is likely that the attending physician will not have immediate access to that patient's medical records. Unless the patient provides an accurate and current listing of all existing prescriptions, the attending physician could easily prescribe a drug

9

that interferes with or interacts with an existing prescription. A person cannot automatically access his or her medical records for review. This inability to readily access and utilize healthcare information is a serious impediment to quality healthcare and the efficiency of healthcare delivery. Adverse reactions to marketed therapies often go unreported to a central location. As a result, regulatory authorities are forced to make decisions that may have an impact on large patient populations based upon incomplete information. Pharmaceutical companies develop competing drugs in distinct programs that cannot and do not take advantage of what may be mutually beneficial baseline (placebo) information.

In general, healthcare information in the United States is documented primarily via taped dictations and/or on paper. It is estimated, for example, that fewer than 3% of hospitals and doctors in the U.S. maintain accessible electronic personal medical records. This information is essentially unavailable to any party other than the health or research professionals working directly with the patient at the same site. Because the records are paper-based, sharing takes place via mail, courier or fax transmittal. Shouldn't our important medical information be accessible to the appropriate parties and used in ways that facilitate patient care? Surely we can learn something from the financial community in this respect. A few recent reports shed light on the way medical records will be handled in the future.

A 2002 report issued by the National Academy of Sciences predicts that during this decade, the new "standard" of healthcare will be digitized, secure and Internet-accessible records, much as financial firms and electronic retailers conduct transactions today. In addition, the Medical Records Institute (MRI) holds an annual conference entitled "Toward an Electronic Patient Record" (www.medrecinst.com/media/document/summary.shtml August 16, 2002). According to a recent report on healthcare documentation, having information that is able to be shared, accessed and accurate is a prerequisite for good healthcare. Having illegible handwriting and other existing documentation practices compromises patient safety and healthcare costs. Clinical research and outcomes analysis are adversely affected by a lack of uniform information capture that is needed to facilitate the derivation of data from routine patient care documentation.

Key principles identified in the MRI report to improve healthcare documentation and make it effective in ensuring quality healthcare are the following:

- Unique patient identification must be assured within and across healthcare documentation systems.

- healthcare documentation must be:
  - Accurate and consistent
  - Complete
  - Timely
  - Interoperable across types of documentation systems
  - Accessible at any time and any place where patient care is needed
  - Auditable
- Confidential and secure authentication and accountability must be provided.

These principles are not unlike those we must apply to clinical research. However, today there is limited to no overlap among the interests of healthcare delivery, basic research and clinical trials. Few or no data are interchanged among these arenas, even on a delayed basis. More remarkably, there is limited and slow data interchange within each of the three arenas, since much of the information is still captured primarily on paper. There are also diverse stakeholders—ranging from physicians and investigators to pharmaceutical company representatives, technology providers to institutional review boards, clinical laboratories, and insurance companies—all of which largely fail to share information. The current situation is illustrated in Figure 1.

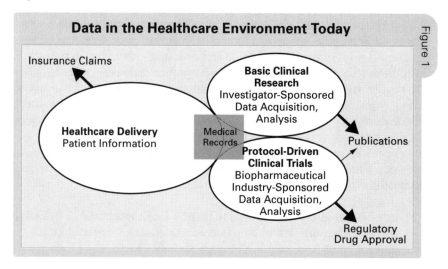

It is unrealistic to think that the entire healthcare industry is going to move rapidly to a paperless delivery system. However, it is not unreasonable to think that benefits of data accessibility can be more quickly accrued in selected areas and that the work can be conducted in a fashion that facilitates future sharing of data. Clinical trial conduct is a prime candidate for such improvement.

Clinical Trials—A Place to Begin

Clinical trials are the most expensive (labor and financial costs) and time-consuming stages in the process of drug development. Later phase programs (e.g., phase III and IV trials), in particular, require extensive oversight and large numbers of study monitors, investigative sites and patient participants. It is widely accepted that eClinical technologies will have the most immediate and noticeable impact on drug development by streamlining clinical trials.

This book explores, in depth, the application of new technologies and redesigned processes to streamline clinical trials. An eClinical trial must encompass not only the implementation of new technology, but also the process modifications and other endeavors that are necessary to leverage the technology and truly reap its benefits. This concept is consistent with the definition of the eClinical trial [eCT] put forth by the Clinical Data Interchange Standards Consortium [CDISC]:

> *A clinical trial in which primarily electronic processes are used to plan, collect (acquire), access, exchange and archive data required for conduct, management, analysis and reporting of the trial.*

eClinical methodology is essentially about increasing information sharing and access to real-time data within and among healthcare delivery systems, basic clinical research and protocol-driven clinical trials. Creating higher levels of information sharing and exchange—from bench to bedside and from research to clinical practice—introduces numerous opportunities to benefit by, and build upon, our knowledge of disease and its progression, of new treatments and individual responses to those treatments. Ultimately, information accessibility and flow will improve the safety and well-being of patients.

There are many positive outcomes that will result from the appropriate use of eClinical methodology to streamline the drug development and approval processes. Among these outcomes are the following:

1. Improve rapid access to clinical trial and clinical research data to facilitate early decisions around the safety and efficacy of investigational interventions.
2. Streamline development functions and reduce direct development costs. Ultimately, this should lower drug prices for consumers, purchasers and payors.
3. Accelerate cycle times, thus shortening the time to market in order to provide new therapies to patients faster and generate prescription sales sooner.
4. Improve access to patient records, for appropriate purposes, while maintaining security and patient privacy.

5. Facilitate the translation of information learned in basic research and clinical trials into clinical practice. As a result, community- and practice-based physicians will have faster access to critical information that will assist them in shaping treatment regimens for their patients. Ultimately, a more efficient translational process will result in more informed, safer and more cost-effective drug utilization.

The next chapter describes today's clinical trials process, heavily dependent on paper, with select enhancements through technology. We view many of these technologies as "point solutions" that streamline specific aspects of the process. Some solutions integrate a number of aspects of clinical trials, but not the entire process.

Chapter 3 presents a vision for clinical trials in the future, emphasizing the difference between the optimal eClinical trial and current solutions that involve the addition of one or more new technologies to long established standard operating processes. The objectives for eClinical trials are described in detail. It is our hope that this vision will play an important role in shaping expectations around the design, use and coordination of eClinical trials technologies.

Chapter 4 introduces an approach to redesigning development processes in order to best evaluate and leverage new technologies. It also includes metrics to compare new technologies and an overview of existing new technologies.

Chapter 5 provides a method for actually implementing the new processes and criteria for selecting technologies for eClinical trials. This sets the stage for subsequent chapters containing details for the execution and evaluation of eClinical trials.

The last five chapters are concerned with the topics of: metrics; regulations; data quality and data integrity; safety surveillance; and the value of industry data standards, with respect to conducting eClinical trials.

The value of easily sharing clinical research information across distinct spheres of our healthcare system is a key area of contention as it not only has an impact on the drug development process, but—ultimately—positively affects the quality of patient care. The sharing of information is becoming more feasible as we uncover better means of addressing patient privacy and confidentiality, while breaking down the barriers that once prevented collaboration and coordination. Stakeholders involved in health-related research and practice now recognize that certain processes, once considered to be a competitive advantage, are inhibiting progress and scientific advancement. This recognition has facilitated the development of industry-wide data interchange standards.

The time and cost of the current clinical development process is unacceptable. We must conduct human research to bring useful new drugs and research results to the public sooner. The need for change is clear. The way that this change occurs is elusive and opaque. The interests of various stakeholders are not aligned.

As the new generation become physicians, clinical researchers and study coordinators, they will have been raised during a time of unprecedented home computer use, and many of the cultural issues we deal with today will be diminished or nonexistent. As we continue to improve the way we plan for and implement eCTs, we must keep our goals in mind and ensure that we pave the way for linking healthcare and clinical research.

This decade poses enormous challenges and opportunities for those of us actively involved in the clinical research industry. eClinical trials represent a significant and profound step in meeting those challenges.

CHAPTER

Today's Clinical Trial

Objectives

- Describe the seven major steps or areas of activity in a typical clinical trial
- Give four examples of technology that have been used to improve the clinical trial process
- Describe four industry-wide issues that remain to be addressed to improve the way we do clinical trials industry-wide

Introduction

From discovery through regulatory approval, clinical trials are the most time consuming and costly aspect of bringing a new therapy to market. Until we can streamline the clinical trials process, development of a new therapy will continue to take approximately a decade and cost more than half a billion dollars. Today, more than 90% of the clinical trials conducted use a paper-based process, which is resource-intensive and does not allow those involved to have accurate information at their fingertips when they need it.

Efforts to add technology to the current clinical trial process have involved many point solutions, which address a specific aspect of a clinical trial. This chapter will explore what constitutes a typical clinical trial today and what progress has been made to apply technology to improve clinical trial conduct.

The Clinical Research Cycle—Paper-Based

The clinical research cycle is made up of distinct areas of activity, which follow the generation of the research hypothesis:

- protocol development
- investigator/site selection and trial preparation (including IRB approval and test article receipt)
- enrollment of subjects and subject participation
- collection, monitoring and processing of data
- clinical trial management
- data analysis and reporting of results
- submission for review by a regulatory agency

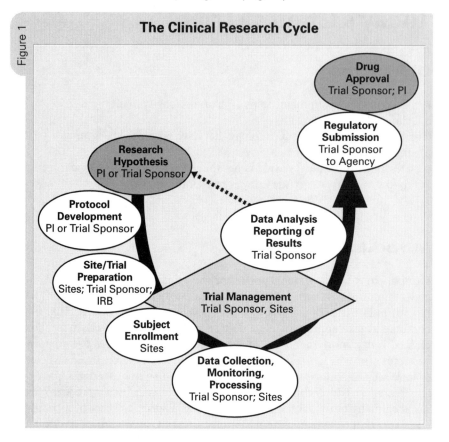

The Clinical Research Cycle

Figure 1

The six distinct areas of activities following the research hypothesis (protocol development through data analysis and reporting of results) constitute a clinical trial. Once the trial is complete, a new hypothesis may be generated, followed by another clinical trial until sufficient supporting data are accumulated. The results of multiple trials, combined with additional information, such as manufacturing and pre-clinical results, are then submitted to a regulatory agency as a submission for review and eventual marketing approval. The graphic in Figure 1 illustrates this cycle:

Protocol Development

The protocol is the plan that specifies the clinical question(s) to be tested and methodologies for statistical evaluation of the results, and also provides a set of instructions for investigative site personnel to follow when a subject is enrolled in a clinical trial. It is common for protocol development to take many months from the development of the initial research hypothesis to final approval by an institutional review board. It is often hard to know ahead of time just how difficult it will be to recruit appropriate subjects or how many subjects will be required to show statistically significant results.

Investigator/Site Selection and Trial Preparation

The selection and preparation of investigators and investigative sites for a clinical trial is another critical step. Once the sites are selected and before a subject can participate, there are a number of documents that must be prepared, signed, approved and maintained on file. Today, these documents are most frequently in notebook binders in paper form. Monitors must ensure, that the investigator's and sponsor's binders or files match and are up to date.

Subject Identification and Enrollment

The identification and evaluation of appropriate subjects to enroll in a trial takes several steps. These include reviewing their medical records to determine whether they are eligible, conducting phone interviews (pre-screening) or performing screening procedures at a visit and/or conducting laboratory tests to ensure that they qualify for the trial. In addition, the subject must go through the informed consent process, which can take anywhere from a few hours to a week or so. The rate at which the subjects are recruited/enrolled plus the time a subject must participate in the trial drive the timeline with respect to availability of the results.

Collection, Monitoring and Processing of Data

Once subjects have signed the informed consent form and are enrolled in the trial, they can undergo screenings and clinical trial procedures. The data gathered from these screenings and procedures are then collected for eventual analysis and inclusion in the study report—which ultimately becomes part of the New Drug Application (NDA) or regulatory submission. The collection and processing of clinical trial data can be labor-intensive, which is one reason investigative sites often think twice about participating in a clinical trial.

Clinical researchers must document patient visits in the medical chart or medical record. A source document represents the first documentation of information pertaining to clinical trials. According to the International Committee on Harmonisation (ICH), source data comprise "…all information in original records and certified copies of original records of clinical findings, observations, or other activities in a clinical trial necessary for the reconstruction and evaluation of the trial. Source data are contained in source documents." Source documents are typically in paper form today, but can also include laboratory results, ECGs and X-rays.

The data are typically transcribed from the source document onto the paper case report forms (CRFs) provided by the sponsor of the trial. The sponsor can be a biotechnology, device manufacturer or pharmaceutical company. CRFs, with three or four NCR (no carbon required) copies per page, are compiled in a casebook.

> **Note**
>
> Note that in some clinical trials a site may enter much of the same information as many as four times. The site initially collects the information onto the chart and/or a source document checklist provided by a CRO or sponsor. The site next enters the data onto the CRF. Then, sites conducting multiple clinical trials often enter selected data into a tracking database to track subject contact and background information, enrollment, visit dates and revenue recognition.

The clinical trial CRF data collected at the investigative site are reviewed by a monitor or clinical research associate (CRA) representing the sponsor company. They ensure that the data are consistent with the source documents, verify that the subjects are real individuals, and that the data are complete, valid, accurate, legible and logical. Monitors compare the data on paper CRFs to paper source documents by hand. The monitor typically handwrites queries onto a separate query resolution page for the site to answer. Because the source documents and CRF data are paper-based, this monitoring takes place at the investigative site.

Figure 2

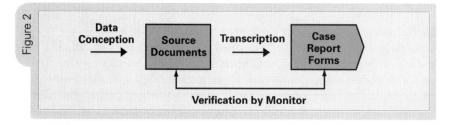

The casebooks are then transferred to the sponsor company or to a contract research organization (CRO). One copy of the casebook, typically the back NCR copy (the least legible), is left at the investigative site.

When sponsor companies or CROs receive a paper CRF, they first follow a login process to acknowledge receipt of the data. There are many ways to do the login, including entry of a date and page identifier by hand into a tracking system or reading bar codes on the CRF. Frequently, there are two or three copies of each CRF page that arrive at the sponsor. After login, one copy is usually filed as an original, while another working copy is sent on for data entry.

Sometimes there is an internal data review or preparation process, after which the sponsor or CRO then enter the data into an operational database that has been developed for that trial. Typically the data are entered twice by two different individuals into two separate but identical databases. The two databases are then compared in order to identify any discrepancies or data entry errors. Any data that do not match are then corrected from a careful review of the paper CRFs. This process results in a single, consistent database of the clinical trial data.

Once the data are in the database, computerized edit checks are run on the data to identify errors that are illogical (e.g., a birthdate with the current year). For most protocols, 70% to 80% of errors caught during data entry or by computerized edit checks are due to missing values, illegible entries or illogical dates. Some data clarifications are not actually errors; rather, the data may just not "fit" into the database the way the database was developed (e.g., weights in pounds rather than kilograms). Monitors or data managers may identify data that need clarification or correction by manually reviewing listings or reports that show lists of the data in printed tables.

When the monitor identifies a data query or discrepancy or error, it must be clarified/corrected so that the data on the source documents and in the casebook at the investigative site and at the sponsor company match the data in the database at the end of the trial (data cleaning). During and at the end of the trial, the investigator must acknowledge that the data are accurate and valid (data verification). The data cleaning and verification processes differ from company to company. Variations may involve documenting all corrections on data clarification/corrections forms (DCFs) at the site, or faxing or sending copies to the site to sign. Once the initial data are recorded, all subsequent data changes must be traceable through an audit trail.

Monitors and data managers have different purposes in mind. The monitor is thinking about the patient and the site and whether the protocol is being followed. Data managers must think about how they are going to get the data into a particular place in the database so that it will end up being "analyzable" and not lost in a comment that no one will ever read.

Note

The CRFs and DCFs are simply paper tools sponsors and CROs use to ensure that source documents match the final database. The ultimate goal is to have the data in the database, report and regulatory submission match the data in the source documents.

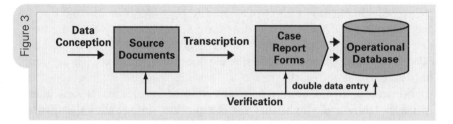

There may also be a reconciliation step to ensure that all of the adverse events match, between the database where they are tracked and the final operational database. There may also be issues with the lab data that must be resolved.

Once all the data are in the database and there are no more outstanding data clarifications, samples of the data are taken for quality assurance purposes to make sure that they are traceable and sufficiently accurate. An audit of the final database is performed against the in-house modified CRF. If more than a minimal number of discrepancies are noted (often 0.5% or more), an entire set of data may need to be re-entered. This can lead to extended delays at the completion of the clinical trial.

Clean vs. "Dirty" Data

Clean vs. dirty data is something that data management grapples with constantly. Should we just get the sites to provide the data as soon as possible, enter it into a computer as it comes and then clean it up? Or, should we wait until the monitor reviews it, has it corrected at the site and then transfers it in-house? One way provides earlier data access, but are the data sufficiently accurate to base decisions on? The other way delays the data access even more.

If or when a QC/QA procedure (e.g. CRF-to-database audit) shows the data in the operational database are complete and accurate within an acceptable error rate, then the database can be locked. The real validation, however, is that the operational database should match the source documents. Unfortunately, this audit is often not performed in finalizing a database. The initial source document verification performed by monitors is assumed to be accurate. Thus, the final database can "drift" from the initial recorded source document, leading to regulatory concerns if and when these discrepancies are uncovered.

Note

Archiving the data and trial-related documentation must occur at the sites and at the sponsor after the trial is over. This entails finding a place for boxes of case report forms to reside, one where they are accessible if an auditor wishes to review them and where they are protected from premature destruction or loss (21 CFR 51.32).

Data Analysis and Reporting

At the point when the database is locked, the statisticians can then break the blind, if the study is a blinded trial, and analyze the results. The statisticians produce tables and graphs that are incorporated into a clinical/statistical report, along with clinical interpretations of the results of the trial. The regulatory submission is a compilation of such reports and other information on the drug and how it is produced/manufactured.

Non-Value-Added Time

The time between when the last subject completes the trial (and the last piece of data is entered in the CRF) and the time the database is locked is "non-value-added time." During this time results cannot be analyzed. The time to database lock is critical because cleaning data adds time and money costs to overall drug development costs. Standard goals for time to database lock range from four to twelve weeks. For some trials, it can last for months.

Clinical Trial Management

Project management in clinical drug development presents singular challenges, including those listed below:

a. Protocol-driven research is unpredictable; the design of each protocol is unique and the design of the protocol may depend on the results of the protocol used in prior clinical trials on that test article.
b. Drug development projects often have a distributed, or decentralized, nature, extending across state and country boundaries and institutions, which results in loss of control by the sponsor.
c. Clinical research projects do not always have coordinated processes working in harmony to ensure smooth trial conduct, and they are not always logically sequential.
d. Development of a drug may take eight to twelve years, which is longer than many clinical project managers hold their positions.
e. Clinical research is a regulated industry with the ultimate customer of the product (data/reports) being a regulatory agency.

Obtaining data and information from the trials is usually not possible in real time—especially with a paper process and a widely distributed project. Hence, the clinical project manager often bases decisions upon outdated information or information that is not compiled in a readily comprehensible form. In a paper-based process, the investigative sites typically report tracking information, such as how many patients they have enrolled in a trial during a week, to the sponsor via phone or fax. This information is then typically entered into a project management system at the central location. The clinical project manager gathers this information (separately from the data coming in on CRFs) in order to follow the status of the project in a more timely manner. The CRF information may not be available to the project manager until weeks after it is entered into the CRF.

Note

Data Access in Global Trials

In paper-based global trials, with sites enrolling subjects in different countries around the world, it can take weeks or even a month to collect the enrollment updates from all of the sites and compile them. This means that, because sponsors do not have the enrollment status, the trial enrollment could continue for weeks longer than needed. The sponsor in such cases would bear the expense of the extra patients enrolled, in time and funding, and many more patients than were necessary could risk exposure to an investigational drug.

In addition, it is typical that adverse events or other safety information is tracked in a separate database. Financial data on the trial budget are never mixed with the clinical information. Thus, the clinical trial project manager may well be dealing with four disparate databases of information that are required to adequately track project status. The site may also keep a management database to track their patients and revenue. Figure 4, which builds on figures 2 and 3 on pages 18 and 20, respectively, shows different databases or documents where much of the same information is entered separately, over and over again.

Figure 4

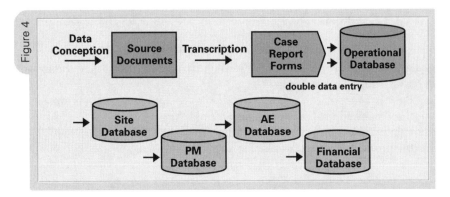

Regulatory Submission, Review and Approval

All of the information on the test drug, including its manufacturing processes, pre-clinical study results, and clinical trial results is compiled into a regulatory submission, which is called a New Drug Application (NDA) in the U.S. [or a Biologic License Application (BLA) for a new biologic therapy or PMA (Product Marketing Application) for a new device]. Currently, these submissions contain volumes of paper (even filling a moving van) and they may take 1 to 3 years to review. The submissions are reviewed by physicians, scientists and statisticians at regulatory agencies, such as the FDA in the U.S. and analogous agencies in Asia and Europe.

The Clinical Research Cycle—The Technology That Can Be Applied Today

Technology can be, and is, leveraged to improve the processes described in the previous section for each of the major activities of a clinical trial. In many cases, this has resulted in improvement in these specific activities, albeit not to the overall clinical trial process. A look at the current state of technology as applied to each of the major activities of a clinical trial is described below.

Protocol Development

Most protocols are developed through word processing or document management systems that facilitate reviews and edits by different team members. Unfortunately, cut and paste methodologies are in use, and desktop word processing is often the only control over the design and development of new protocols. The use of more sophisticated document management tools can help in organizing and standardizing the process of protocol development.

There are other technologies that support protocol development on a clinical trial. For example, technology is now available to simulate trials as they are being designed to determine whether they would be effective in determining safety and efficacy, based upon estimates and metrics from similar trials conducted previously. Another type of newly available technology simulates biochemical pathways in the body and can be used to predict and model outcomes of drug therapies. Using these applications can help improve the design of the trials before they are initiated so that the protocol may be more realistic or the study will have a better chance of detecting true treatment differences.

Yet another recent tool is the use of software applications for protocol authoring/modeling, which in this case means that the protocol would be broken down into steps with algorithms that could help optimize study design when developing a protocol and set the stage for database development. These tools can help identify inconsistencies in protocol design and can prevent costly amendments and modifications to the protocol during the conduct of the study.

Unfortunately, streamlining protocol development hinges on improving the team interactions and the review and approval procedures within companies. These various stakeholders need to be able to reach agreement or consensus and make decisions quickly in order to finalize the protocol. Technology is not the total solution. Technology can help, but delays in protocol development are often primarily a process issue.

Investigator/Site Selection and Trial Preparation

Other than spreadsheets, technology has been applied sparingly to the site preparation of the trial process. There are usually in-house systems to log dates when the documents required to initiate a trial are completed or approvals are received. These tracking systems, however, require time on the part of an individual, such as a monitor or project assistant, to communicate with sites and log these dates. Sites may keep a similar tracking system themselves. This centralizing and communicating may also involve compiling a database with information about the investigators/sites that enables the selection of appropriate sites to conduct the trial. The Internet is also proving to be a useful communication tool for connecting sites with trials and vice versa.

> **Note**
>
> **Paper in the IRB Process**
> In a trial with multiple sites, some of the sites will be able to use a central IRB, but others will need to use the IRB affiliated with their institution. There may be as many versions of an IRB submission or informed consent form as there are IRBs. Today, this means a tremendous amount of faxing or express mailings to obtain IRB review and approval. One way technology can help is by eliminating the amount of faxing and mailing; if IRBs were to use an electronic process with workflow and electronic signatures, they could save substantial paper and time.

Enrollment of Subjects

With respect to subject recruitment, several options for technology exist. Communication is a key issue; for example, potential subjects can learn about the trial from their practicing physician, from advertisements through different media (television, radio, newspapers, direct mail campaigns) or by searching the Internet. If a trial is a large one, there may even be an outsourcing component to a central call center, where calls are fielded from potential subjects and candidates are referred to appropriate sites.

Many sites have contact/recruitment databases or a type of study management database to consolidate information on their potential clinical trial subjects, follow their existing trial subjects and track their revenue based upon progress of the subjects on trials.

The sites often collect demographics, medical history information, visit dates and other data in their recruitment databases and/or through their screening procedures. These data are then typically re-entered into the CRF when a subject is enrolled in a trial. Consequently, such tools and databases are typically only used for the purposes of the site personnel.

Collection, Monitoring and Processing of Data

In a paper-based process, CRFs typically have three or four NCR copies per page, and the monitoring is typically done by hand at the investigative site comparing CRF data with source documents. The CRF data are later entered twice at a central location into a database. Such a database may be a proprietary system, or it may be a commercial application that supports the "back-end" data management process. Such systems are referred to as Clinical Data Management Systems (CDMS) or similar terms. These back-end systems typically support edit checking, query resolution, audit trails and other data management activities at the sponsor or CRO.

Over the past fifteen to twenty years, many different forms of site-based capture of clinical trial data have been developed. Data collection technology that has been applied to improve clinical trial data collection is generally referred to as electronic data capture (EDC). EDC is defined by the Clinical Data Interchange Standards Consortium (CDISC) as:

Collecting or acquiring data as a permanent electronic record with or without a human interface (e.g., using data collection systems or applications that are modem-based, web-based, optical mark/character recognition, or involve audio text, interactive voice response, graphical interfaces, clinical laboratory interfaces, or touch screens). Note: "Permanent" in the context of these definitions implies that any changes made to the electronic data are recorded via an audit trail.

First Generation EDC Tools

The first attempts to improve the paper-based process involved data collection technology such as facsimile; optical mark recognition (OMR), which is used to correct standardized school tests; or optical character recognition (OCR). The combination of facsimile and OCR can have significant impact on selected trials, but it does not provide a general purpose solution to the data collection issue. More specifically, the use of facsimile actually adds work for the site personnel and does not reduce the amount of paper. OCR and OMR are not yet adequate to allow for the accurate recognition of free-form text and are therefore of value only for certain types of clinical trials, e.g., post-marketing trials.

Remote Data Entry (RDE). The first computer-based EDC implementations involved proprietary systems, made up of a computer and pre-loaded software specific to the conduct of a single clinical research project and deployed at investigative sites. These computers could only be used for the purpose of that protocol, and no additional software was to be installed and run on them. When data were entered into such computers, they were stored locally at the site until the user connected (e.g., through a dial-up connection) to transfer the data to the sponsor. At the end of the research project, the computer was usually removed from the physician's office. If a physician chose to participate in multiple research projects with multiple sponsors, multiple proprietary computer systems were required. It became a problem for a very active research site to allocate enough physical space to accommodate all the computers, not to mention keep the software applications straight.

The earliest systems involved nothing more than the collection of data from the site, with simple data edit checks to improve the quality of the data. The data were moved directly into traditional CDMS solutions, and data review, data quality checks and monitoring were performed manually through the CDMS and locally at the site. The system was nothing more than a data entry tool.

If there were edit checks built into the data entry application at the site, then the principal benefit of RDE was that it could result in improved quality of the data submitted. If the sites entered the data and transferred it shortly after collection, this strategy could also expedite the availability of data and improve study management. Users obtained fast data entry performance because they were running a local application, but local maintenance, validation and security issues caused RDE to fall into disfavor. (See Chapter 7.

A variation of RDE is that some companies have the monitors (not the site personnel) enter data at the sites. This moves data entry from the central sponsor site to the local investigative site. However, data entry must wait for monitoring visits, and all the advantages of feedback to the site personnel through data entry were lost.

Interactive Voice Response Systems. Interactive Voice Response Systems (IVRS), which have been used in clinical trials for more than ten years, are another first generation EDC tool. An IVRS, historically, is an interactive speech or touch-pad menu-driven system that takes the caller through a series of prompts. Callers then respond to questions by pressing buttons on the phone keypad. Most uses of IVRS are in the consumer and customer support area in financial, retail or other commercial areas. IVRS are typically used for clinical trials in select areas such as patient randomization, adverse event reporting, drug supply management, tracking visit milestones, assisting with study startup or collecting subject diary information.

A key feature of IVRS is that any site with access to a telephone can use it. In addition, IVRS can support multiple languages, operate automatically 24 hours a day and provide real-time access to a database without a computer network. However, the amount of data that a site can transfer via IVRS is limited by the interface itself. It will not expand beyond its present use until IVRS technology improves in areas such as voice recognition, text-to-speech and web integration.

Second Generation EDC

The benefits of today's EDC applications go far beyond simple data capture. Although some of the first generation EDC tools were little more than data entry applications, the concept has evolved significantly over the past ten years. First generation EDC tools are still in use today for specific purposes (e.g., IVRS for randomization), but second generation EDC applications available today are likely to contain significant, integrated functionality that allows much more of the clinical trial process to be managed electronically. These EDC solutions have sophisticated data checks that can be applied across pages, visits and even patients in a clinical trial. The current crop of second generation EDC solutions can provide data access for systematic review and allow manual queries by all of the sponsor personnel responsible for data review.

Although it is possible to directly enter data into the EDC application (known as eSource and discussed in detail in Chapter 3), most sponsors currently use EDC applications with traditional paper-based source documents. The EDC applications typically track the process of source document verification, as well as in-house data reviews. Finally, EDC can track and document electronic signatures by site and sponsor personnel.

The advantages of EDC applications over paper-based clinical trials are numerous. First, as data are entered, automated data edit checks alert the investigative site to possible errors in data entry. The site can check while the source document is readily available, rather than months later in a typical paper-based process. This immediate feedback can not only help the site in correcting the initial issue but can help educate the site to avoid the error in the future. Since there is no delay as is typical in the paper process, costly errors can be avoided much earlier in the process.

Second, the EDC applications allow sponsors to review and evaluate the data as soon as they are entered. This immediate access to data is one of the major advantages to the sponsor and represents an area where patient safety in clinical trials can be improved. The sponsor can also determine if data entry is tardy (in relation to the date it was collected) and can automatically track and review the quality of the data. Since many activities are performed through the EDC application (entry, review, editing, locking), it is possible to track and semi-automate the completion of these activities. EDC has been shown to shorten the non-value-added time between when all of the subject data are available (all subjects have completed the trial) and the point of the database lock.

In addition, since many activities are performed through the EDC tool, it is possible to collect and analyze metrics about personnel performance, resolution of queries, source document verification and other trial activities. This operational information is very valuable in improving the efficiency of the clinical trial process.

EDC alone does not bring quality improvement, cost control and time-liness to clinical trials. It is essential that the company that implements EDC also fully evaluate their process and the ways that EDC applications change the process. Only by re-engineering the process can the sponsor realize the potential of EDC. (See Chapter 4.)

EDC Architectures

The EDC solutions discussed thus far consist of both decentralized and centralized systems. In the case of decentralized systems, the software solution, and frequently the hardware, is provided to a physician's practice and then used outside the direct control of the software vendor or study sponsor. These systems have inherent disadvantages because the physician's staff has to set up and maintain the proprietary system. The systems also require more support from the vendor due to the decentralized environment. Finally, when local hardware/software is present at the site, the FDA guidelines require a set of local Standard Operating Procedures (SOPs) to provide for validation, security, backup and local control of the application and data.

In an attempt to ease system management and regulatory problems in a decentralized environment, some vendors introduced second generation systems that offer centralized clinical trial solutions. These solutions do not require any specific hardware, and they do not store any application software or data locally on the computer. They typically use a standard browser as the interface, and the Internet as the medium for transferring data. This eliminates the necessity to store information at the sites and makes system management and regulatory compliance much easier. The application and database are typically housed in a secure facility where redundant power, Internet access and security procedures can ensure maximal availability and security of data.

Regardless of where the clinical data are stored—site computer or centralized repository—it is essential that appropriate measures are in place to prevent unauthorized changes to the data. These measures could include the use of a trusted third party, digital notary and other accepted techniques to ensure data integrity.

As of this writing, broadband, high bandwidth data transfer is not available at many investigative sites. Therefore, online applications must be designed to work effectively over dial-up connections. This limitation means that data entry processes must be carefully designed, and some high bandwidth data transfer (e.g., MRI or CT data) may not be practically transferred. (When high bandwidth or broadband connections are more widely available, online data collection applications can offer much more functionality.)

Another second generation EDC system in use is known as a hybrid system. There are many variations of hybrid systems, some with local applications but a central database, others with both local and central databases. For hybrid applications with local databases, the site can work either online or offline. If the user is working offline, the system stores the data on that computer until it makes an Internet or dial-up connection, at which point the data transfers to the sponsor. If the user is working online, the data transfers during the session.

On the surface, offline or hybrid systems may appear to have some advantages over online systems, because they appear to provide the benefits of online systems without requiring constant connectivity. However, operating an offline system does drive up the overall complexity of the data collection effort and can compromise some of the potential benefits of electronic data collection. Once data are stored outside of a central, secure facility the possibility of database corruption and loss is significantly increased. Sites may also not choose to transfer data immediately, and the overall timeliness of the data and potential for intervention drops. Supporting this increase in complexity falls mainly on the vendor deploying the solution, but the end user must support the software application running locally. The issues of system validation and local SOPs are the same as those used for the aforementioned distributed systems. Most agree that the ultimate solution to clinical trial data collection involves a completely online system with no local data storage. However, for the online solution to work, users involved in data entry will need guaranteed access to the application. This guaranteed access implies redundancy in the connection between the user's computer and the host system.

Early data collection systems were based almost exclusively on personal computers (desktops or notebooks) as the user input device. But subjects of clinical trials have now begun to use newer handheld devices such as personal digital assistants (PDAs), and researchers are using tablet computers. Several companies offer PDAs to replace the paper-based diaries subjects use in some clinical trials. Today, these PDAs typically operate in offline mode, although in the future many of these will likely operate by wireless data transfer. The PDA stores the clinical data until it can be transferred to the study database. In this case, the data entered into the PDA are the source data, and all the issues associated with using an offline device for source data collection must be addressed.

Most recently, with the convergence of handheld computers with cellular telephones, there has been substantial interest and early use of systems that involve simple EDC through a cell phone and/or a handheld computer with cellular access. In the long run, this type of data collection, especially for patient diaries, is likely to be a predominant data entry format.

A list of the strategies for data acquisition, along with variations in techniques that have been used, can be found in Table 1.

Integrated EDC Tools

EDC continues to evolve. A handful of the leading vendors have integrated their EDC tools with their own or other clinical data management systems. In doing so, the vendors have taken a step closer to optimizing the eClinical trial. These systems allow the sponsor to use libraries of forms and tradi-

Table 1

Data Collection Strategies With Varying Techniques

Strategy	Variations
First Generation EDC	■ Optical mark recognition and optical character recognition (paper data collection and computer read). ■ Interactive Voice Response Systems ■ Offline data collection using a PC at the site, followed by point-to-point transfer to a central computer. ■ Offline data collection via handheld devices with point-to-point transfer to a central computer.
Second Generation EDC	■ Online data collection, monitoring and processing through Internet connectivity to a secure central database. ■ Hybrid systems with two modes of operation—online data collection via the Internet without local storage or offline data collection with local storage prior to transfer to a central computer. ■ Enhanced IVRS

tionally hand-entered data along with EDC tools (and in several cases, along with clinical safety reporting systems). The result is a more efficient back-end process for the sponsor and an easier transition from traditional data management to newer electronic technologies. This step, just now being made available, may likely not be visible to the investigative sites involved in the clinical trials, but may yield significant efficiencies.

Most of the data collection tools today do not include features that address the specific needs of sites. Consequently, as mentioned under "Subject Enrollment," the sites often have much of the same data needed for the trial in their own databases for patient recruitment. They typically re-enter these data into the EDC systems.

Data Analysis and Reporting of Results

Statisticians have actually relied on technology for years in order to do their jobs, from statistical analyses to producing results in tables and graphs to help clinicians interpret study findings. The sooner the database is locked, the sooner the statisticians can perform their art. They typically use an application called SAS for the statistical analyses.

The recent improvements in this area have been largely process improvements. Once the statisticians ensure that the protocol has an appropriate statistical design and analysis section, they do not need to wait until the database is locked to do any further work. Instead, they can design the tables they intend to use based upon the data being collected, access test data during the trial to ensure that these "fit" into the tables and do not have spurious values, and basically be prepared to analyze the results as soon as they are available.

Clinical Trial Management

Many companies have developed proprietary tracking systems or have purchased tracking systems developed specifically for this industry. Unfortunately, the concept of "clinical trial management" is interpreted differently by different sponsors and vendors. The result is that the tools available cover a vast array of different functions. Some clinical trial management tools focus on collecting site-specific data and budget information, while others focus on the management of operational aspects of the central data management process. Still others focus on the "program management" aspects of clinical trials. Many times, these systems are referred to as clinical trial management systems (CTMS). In addition, the investigative sites may also be tracking much of this information in their own site management databases. Trial management is an area that needs to be streamlined through earlier access to high quality electronic data. It should not be necessary to enter essentially the same data repeatedly into multiple different databases, with each transcription or data entry point adding another opportunity for a disparity to occur.

When coupled with EDC tools or integrated with new applications, clinical trial management tools can make use of the "metadata," or data about the data—e.g., who submitted the data and when—to automatically collect and analyze operational information about the clinical trial conduct. (See Chapter 6.)

Visualization tools are now available to support data review and project management. Newly developed tools allow project managers, medical reviewers or physician scientists to explore data and be alerted to significant safety events in data through visualization software and algorithms designed to capture rare and important events. Although traditional data exploration has not been viewed favorably in the industry, these new tools can reveal important trends and allow for the development of new hypotheses to be further tested in clinical trials. Other visualization tools simply make the data easier to review in the sense that a picture is worth a thousand words. The FDA is using certain of these for data review.

Regulatory Submission, Review and Approval for Marketing

Ten years ago, the FDA paved the way for electronic submission of clinical trials data and regulatory submissions through the Computer Assisted NDA (CANDA) process. Pharmaceutical companies saw an opportunity to speed approval and complied with a vengeance—NDAs were accompanied by electronic submissions produced on proprietary systems that were installed on the desktop of FDA reviewers. Unfortunately, the standards for the CANDA were loose, and the profusion of different systems was unworkable for the FDA. Beginning in 1997, the FDA provided guidance documents to allow the electronic submission of data in a standards-based manner. Guidance documents on standard electronic submissions could dramatically facilitate their reviews, particularly if data standards were used. (See Chapter 10.) In addition, receipt of electronic data in standard formats would allow them to view data across submissions within a given therapeu-

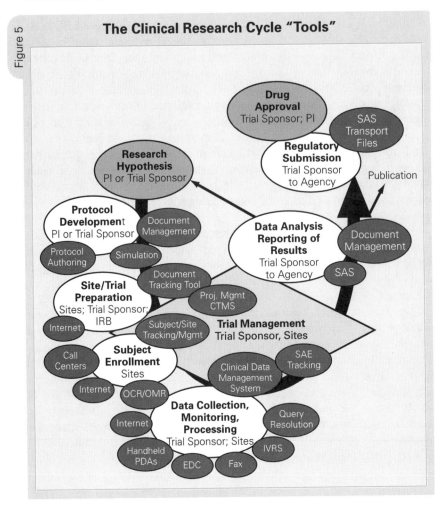

Figure 5

The Clinical Research Cycle "Tools"

tic area. This could, in turn, facilitate reviews and/or potentially decrease the number of patients required for placebo-controlled studies. Electronic submissions would also allow the reviewers to subset data or review the analyses that were done without going back to the sponsor to provide additional analyses. The current FDA requirement for receipt of electronic data is in a form called SAS transport files. They also accept documents in electronic form, through the portable document format (pdf). There are efforts to standardize the structures and content of the data they receive, and the FDA is also collaborating in the development of review tools. All of these steps are subordinate to the overall goal to facilitate and improve their review process. Chapter 10 provides more details on clinical data interchange standards.

Figure 5 illustrates how the various tools mentioned above correspond to the distinct areas of activity within the clinical research cycle.

In looking at figure 5, it is clear that the attempts to date to improve the paper-based process have centered on applying technology to improve specific aspects of the clinical trial process (e.g., protocol development, investigator selection, subject recruitment, data collection, document tracking, clinical trial management). In general, the desire has been to decrease the time required to accomplish a specific activity (a point solution)—not optimizing the entire process.

Unfortunately, the result of these point-based applications is to produce "islands" of information and data. There is often no guarantee that data collected in one application can be easily exported or imported by other applications. These data are often redundant, sometimes inconsistent and not readily available. Consequently, its intrinsic value is compromised.

To gain full benefit from new technology, it is essential that a much higher level of integration and standardization be achieved. The discrete solutions available today must be extended and integrated such that all participants in the process benefit.

The Clinical Data Interchange Standards Committee (CDISC) defines an electronic clinical trial (eCT) as:

> *A clinical trial in which primarily electronic processes are used to plan, collect (acquire), access, exchange and archive data required for conduct, management, analysis and reporting of the trial.*

The definition addresses the actual concept of what an eCT is. While electronic data collection (EDC) can address the data collection (acquisition) aspect of a clinical trial, it does not address all the facets of an electronic clinical trial. An electronic clinical trial requires the exchange and archiving of electronic data and also encourages the leveraging of technology for trial planning, management, conduct, analysis, reporting and archiving.

Although there are companies today that have conducted electronic clinical trials, there are few that will state that they have conducted the opti-

eClinical Trial Technologies in Today's Clinical Studies

The vast majority of biopharmaceutical companies and contract research organizations (CROs) view eClinical technologies as critical to their long-term development strategies. And eClinical technology adoption is clearly rising steadily.

CenterWatch and CDISC jointly conducted an ambitious research project among approximately 750 organizations in 2002. The project examined industry-wide usage, adoption and implementation of new technologies for clinical trials as well as the use of data interchange standards. Four separate surveys—for biopharmaceutical companies; CRO/service providers; investigative sites; and technology providers/ EDC vendors—were distributed. Several major professional organizations including the Drug Information Association, the Association of Clinical Research Professionals and the Association of American Medical Colleges assisted in disseminating these surveys.

The results indicate that sponsors and CROs are using eClinical technologies for 24% of their phase I–IV trials—up from only 12% in 2000. Sponsors and CROs anticipate using these technologies for almost half of all clinical projects by 2004. Each sponsor reported that, in 2002, they used eClinical trial technologies on an average of four clinical research studies. Moreover, a high percentage of biopharmaceutical and CRO companies (84%) view eClinical trial technologies as major strategic initiatives to shorten development cycle times and improve data quality.

mal electronic clinical trial. Additional issues that remain in applying technology to streamline the overall clinical trial processes include the following:

- We have not solved the overall problem of streamlining the entire clinical trial process while making quality data available to those who need it as soon as possible.
- The organizational and enterprise-wide changes necessary to truly leverage EDC have not yet been adequate.
- Exchanging data among different systems and entities is tedious, typically requiring extra time at the beginning to design specific databases, or integration techniques at the end of the process.
- Sites may well be using multiple different computer applications concurrently. They may also be re-entering much of the same data multiple times, especially if they have their own management systems in addition to source documents and EDC applications.
- A link has not yet been made between healthcare data and clinical trial data.

Sponsors and CROs do perceive barriers to adopting eClinical technologies at this time. These barriers are largely a function of the relative nascence of EDC and eClinical technology. Sponsor and CRO companies perceive a high level of uncertainty given the absence of clear regulatory direction (e.g., 21 CFR part 11), the need for data interchange standards and a highly fragmented technology provider market. Nearly two-thirds of sponsor companies believe that current eClinical solutions offer inadequate functionality at this time. As such, less than half of sponsors and CROs report having had positive experiences with e-trial technologies to date.

Investigative sites are looking for new approaches to better manage their financial and business operations. The majority—77%—believes that eClinical technologies will play a key role in streamlining study conduct activities and improving operating margins. Half of the 355 investigative sites responding to the survey have had positive experiences with eClinical technologies. Only 25% of investigative sites, however, report having standard operating procedures to accommodate the use of new technology solutions.

Conclusion

The clinical research cycle includes distinct areas of activity, which we have discussed in terms of existing processes as well as technology solutions currently being applied to improve these processes. It is clear that the technology that has been applied has been limited to specific problem areas, and none of the technology has had much impact on reducing redundant data entry or the amount of paper used in trial conduct. The vast majority of clinical trials are still being conducted with a paper-based process. The reasons for this are complex, being related to the wide variation of quality/functionality of existing EDC solutions, real and perceived regulatory risks, inadequate use of data standards and the overall slowness of adoption that is characteristic of the pharmaceutical industry. An electronic clinical trial involves primarily electronic processes. Although this is occurring sporadically today, most would agree that the optimal electronic clinical trial has yet to be conducted.

CHAPTER 3

The Optimal Electronic Clinical Trial—A Vision for the Future

Objectives

- Describe five of the goals that an optimal electronic clinical trial should achieve.
- Define the concepts forming the basis of an optimal electronic clinical trial and how they differ from trials conducted today.

Introduction

To conduct an optimal electronic clinical trial (eCT), one must first adhere to the definition of an electronic clinical trial, which involves primarily electronic processes. In addition, one must go beyond simply adding point solutions for improvement of discrete activities in the clinical trial process. In addition to integrating and improving technologies, significant process redesign must take place. Eventually we must more closely link clinical trials to healthcare. All of the stakeholders in a clinical trial must benefit. The optimal electronic clinical trial is an achievable ideal, but one that realistically will require changes in technology, process, standards and the regulatory environment.

This chapter paints a vision for the optimal electronic clinical trial.

Goals for the Optimal Electronic Clinical Trial

A number of opportunities arise for process improvement when one truly leverages technology. The desired outcome, the true optimal electronic clinical trial (eCT), occurs when implementation of new technology is coupled in the best possible way with redesigned processes (see Chapter 4). If the industry is to achieve an optimal eCT, several goals should be reached. These goals include:

- Built-in Quality
- Facilitation of Site Processes
- Facilitation of Monitoring Processes
- Facilitation of Data Management Processes
- Improved Communication and Coordination
- Improved Project Management
- Standardization

Built-in Quality

One good example of the "built-in quality concept" is from the automobile industry. At one time, the quality resulting from the mass production process was so bad that many automobiles were pulled from the production line and stacked because of problems encountered during the assembly process. Cars that did get shipped tended to have a large number of defects per vehicle. When engineers diagnosed the root cause of the problems and corrected it in real time, quality improved dramatically and the average time to build a car decreased significantly. This result stemmed from application of the Deming philosophy, which was first implemented by the Japanese and applied to the automobile industry. The Japanese automobile manufacturers that successfully embraced the Deming philosophy are still the quality leaders in the automobile industry.

> When should errors be corrected during a clinical trial? Some suggest that personnel should just get the data in faster, regardless of the quality. Others believe that because of the data clarification or query resolution processes, the push for speed will only result in "piles of queries" stacking up at the end of the line—like poor quality automobiles. Errors in data collected may also compromise the work of a safety monitoring review board.
>
> Note

Errors in clinical research may occur at many points: when the study coordinator enters the chart data; when data are transcribed onto the CRF; when the monitor reviews the CRF data and verifies it with the medical chart; or when it goes to the sponsor for entry into the operational database.

These errors may not be detected until statisticians or medical writers get involved. The later the error is found in the process, the longer it takes to correct and the greater the cost (in time, resources and quality).

The graph in Figure 1 shows calculated costs to correct an individual error (query or data clarification) found at different points in the process. Many estimate the cost per query to be approximately $75 to $100 per query, but this amount clearly varies depending on when and where the query is resolved, and it also seems to be an average figure for queries resolved in a batch (as opposed to one that is corrected alone). Even though an error would typically not be corrected as a stand-alone, the message is clear regarding the relationship between cost and point of error detection. If an error is caught in the last QA or by the FDA, ramifications may be more severe than cost alone. Such an error could promote distrust in the rest of the data in the submission by a regulatory reviewer if it is not caught and corrected in advance.

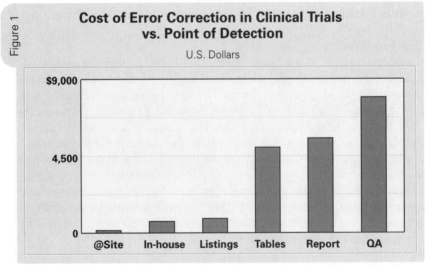

Note: These costs were calculated based upon the cost of personnel hours utilized for the required activities associated with errors/queries detected at different points in the process.

A query does not mean that the data are necessarily wrong. It is possible that the data are simply not entered into the CRF in the format needed for the database. The earlier data coordinators and monitors know how they should collect and document data, the fewer queries or data clarifications will result. The proven approach to effectively reducing the total number of errors is twofold. First, plans must be developed in advance for the database structure, data management procedures and data edit checks to be performed by data management. Second, the way the data should be collected and will be monitored must be communicated to the entire project team (including the site personnel).

Note

Two key messages regarding built-in quality are that:

- The earlier an error is detected, the sooner it can be rectified and the easier and less costly it is to correct.

- In the planning stage of a trial, the way the data will be collected and managed should be decided early and communicated to all involved in collecting, monitoring, and managing the data, regardless of the technology or the process.

Unfortunately, in practice, data may be entered in the medical chart and/or the case report form well after the patient has departed from the visit, which makes recall more difficult and errors more likely. In addition, the monitor and study coordinator may think the data are fine, only to find out that the format is not what the data manager wants. The data managers may not develop the database until after the trial has begun. Or, a high percentage of CRFs may be retrieved with data entered before the first edit checks are run and the areas where data clarifications are needed are identified. To compound the mistake, more and more CRFs are being completed in the same incorrect way at the same time before a root problem is discovered or communicated.

Collecting data electronically (EDC) provides tremendous opportunity for building in quality at the start and making the goals of an optimal electronic clinical trial achievable. Edit checks can be integrated into the data capture front end so that when data are not entered correctly, a message pops up to that effect. The error or query can be resolved as soon as possible, ideally before the study coordinator has time to forget the visit and while the subject is still in the office.

Computers also can automatically record and maintain electronically the time and date of data entry and who was logged into the computer at the time that data were entered. Then if the data are ever changed, this alteration can be documented electronically, including information indicating who changed it at what time and on what date. This creates an automatic audit trail. If maintained properly electronically, it satisfies regulatory requirements for an audit trail of any recording or altering of clinical trial data. This information about the data is called metadata. Metadata is also useful when trying to track information for metrics and for implementing standards, which are discussed in Chapters 6 and 10.

Electronic source documentation (eSource)

New products, such as PDAs, tablet computers and enhanced wireless, facilitate the ability of researchers to collect data initially via electronic data capture. This type of data capture is an example of "eSource," or electronic source documentation. The concept of eSource is very exciting because it eliminates the final source of transcription error and the final source of delay in access to data—the errors and delays that occur in transcription from the source to the CRF. Data can be entered once, preferably at the time of the patient encounter, and be carried through the entire process. In fact, we have been using eSource data for years in clinical trials; despite the fact that laboratory data are printed out on forms, their initial entry is electronic.

To properly understand the definition of eSource data, it is important to first recall the ICH's definition of source data.

> **Source Data:** *All information in original records, certified records, and certified copies of original records of clinical findings; observations; or other activities in a clinical trial necessary for the reconstruction and evaluation of the trial. Source data are contained in source documents (original records or certified copies). [ICH]*

> **eSource Data:** *Source data (per ICH) captured initially into a permanent electronic record.*

> *Note: "Permanent" in the context of this definition implies that any changes made to the electronic data are recorded via an audit trail.*

Realistically, complete eSource data collection may not be possible for many clinical trials. But, in theory, the fewer times researchers enter, transcribe and re-enter data, the lower the probability that they will incur an error due to the process. Even without complete eSource, it would be best if technology eliminated or minimized re-entry of the same data.

During a typical investigative study, there are three or four points when essentially the same data may be entered:

- The medical chart (usually paper but sometimes an electronic medical record).
- A source document checklist or form designed for the trial to ensure that all of the data are collected at a visit.
- A clinical trial record (paper CRF or electronic data capture tool).
- Often the site employs a patient/site tracking tool (e.g., for tracking visits and revenue and for patient databases used for recruitment purposes).

In a paper-based process, these data are then re-entered twice into a database at the sponsor company, site or CRO. In addition, a trial tracking or project management tool at the sponsor site and an adverse event or safety database may raise the number of redundant data entries to six or eight (see Figure 2).

What if technology could make it easier to collect the required data at a subject visit, while tracking this and site management information automatically? Data could then potentially be entered once (e.g., in a recruitment/management database controlled by the site) and replicated through to other places as deemed appropriate (while retaining confidential or subject privacy-related information under the control/view of the sites). What would the data entry illustration look like in this case? (See Figure 3.)

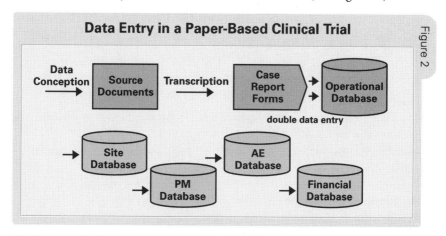

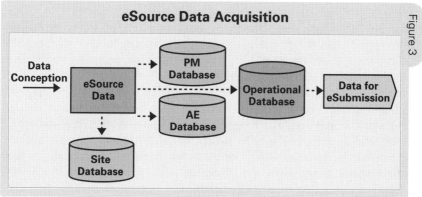

Please note that the eSource data may come from multiple different sources, including clinical laboratory data, ECGs, electronic patient diaries, or other sources.

The eSource vision allows for the electronic collection of a "superset" of data, beyond what is required for the eCRF (i.e., essentially collecting information electronically that may today be collected on paper source documents and in a site tracking database). Therefore, it supports documentation of complete clinical cases in addition to protocol-specific clinical trial (CRF) documentation and would support the distribution of this information to different sources to serve the various necessary purposes, thus eliminating re-entry of the same data multiple times.

Clearly, eSource offers many potential advantages. Most observers of the clinical trial process see that eSource data collection is the best eventual methodology for data collection. However, this eSource vision, while very enticing, presents several challenges.

CDISC-CW Survey

High Preference for eSource Documentation Online

According to the results of the CDISC-CenterWatch research project conducted recently among 750 organizations, there is very high receptivity to eSource documentation online, and there is a high expectation that it will play a critical role in the future. More than two-thirds (70%) of sponsor and CRO companies and three out of four investigative sites believe that eSource documentation online is one of the best ways to leverage new eClinical trial technology.

These are the major issues that remain to be addressed for eSource adoption:

- Regulatory
- Absence of standards
- Clinical and research

One challenge stems from the interpretations of FDA regulations. Perceptions persist that the FDA wants to see paper to verify clinical trial data with a paper back-up. This is simply not true, according to the FDA itself (go to www.fda.gov/cder/regulatory/ersr/default.htm). What the FDA wants to see is a permanent record (electronic or paper) at the investigative site of the first recordings of clinical data regardless of storage medium. In fact, the FDA has been accepting eSource for years—both in medical device trials and in clinical laboratory data. Clinical laboratory data are nothing more than electronically collected data that "seem" like paper because they are printed out onto forms in a physician's office or at a trial sponsor's location. The initial data are actually electronic.

Another regulatory concern with eSource resides in the predicate Good Clinical Practice (GCP) rule that investigators must maintain the case histories they collect. In practice, this means that they must have control of the data. In the electronic world, control could mean physical possession of the database, and the SOPs around access, backup and changes to the database. With online eSource, this cannot exist—the investigator has nothing but a web browser and no physical control of the data. Therefore, the investigator must be able to demonstrate that the database was held by a trusted third party, was under strict control in that setting through software controls, access restrictions, procedures and other security measures. The environment for online eSource therefore requires a good deal of stringency about the systems, the validation of the application (to assure that it doesn't inadvertently change data) and the trustworthiness of the host.

Another challenge is the availability of systems to collect eSource. There are currently at least two plausible approaches for expanding the usage of eSource in clinical trials. One approach would be to modify existing elec-

Regulatory Concerns About the Collection of All Types of Data, Including eSource

Note

The FDA remains steadfast in its concern over the "ALCOA"—attributable, legible, contemporaneous, original and accurate—nature of data, which embody the attributes of data quality. The FDA wants to know that the data they are reviewing represent the data that the investigator collected, whether the data were handled electronically or on paper. In the paper process, the three-part NCR form combined with adherence to standard operating procedures solves this problem—one form is left with the investigator, and the other two are sent in. All changes are documented on data clarification forms or on the CRF itself. As a result, there is a complete audit trail from the original data to the final database. Electronic data must be managed just as stringently. In fact, because electronic data can be changed without an apparent trace, it is even more important to be vigilant about the data. To this end, the FDA developed 21 CFR Part 11 and guidance on this—The Electronic Records/Electronic Signature rule that guides the electronic collection and management of data (see Appendix E and Chapter 7).

tronic medical record (EMR) systems or create a new EMR system that supports clinical trials and complies with all applicable regulations, including 21 CFR 11. Unfortunately, since market penetration of EMR systems in the U.S. is quite small and the growth of usage of such systems is not expected to expand dramatically in the near future, it is not clear that this approach could provide a significant increase in the rate of adoption of eSource. It should be noted that several European countries are far ahead of the U.S. in terms of the availability of suitable systems. A second approach is to modify an existing EDC system or create a new EDC system that is capable of capturing more than just trial information. Sites could use this system not only to conduct clinical trials but also to manage patient visits. Such systems could dramatically increase the usage of eSource, reduce many of the redundant data entry issues and potentially provide real benefit to the sites. In any approach, the applications will need to meet the strict requirements of patient data privacy imposed by the Health Insurance Portability and Accountability Act (HIPAA) and all the relevant electronic clinical trial regulations. In addition, it must be clear that the investigator is in control of the source data.

Another challenge to expanded eSource is the adoption of data interchange standards that support both the healthcare community and the biopharmaceutical industry. Progress being made in this area is covered in Chapter 10.

From a clinical and research perspective, it is imperative that the collection of eSource data does not degrade the clinical workflow or negatively impact the patient/physician interaction. Recent advances in technology are making such systems/technologies more viable, but it is not clear that such an option exists today. An operational issue with eSource is that data must continuously be backed up to prevent permanent data loss due to technology failure. This is an option available today with an ASP model.

Despite all these challenges, the benefits offered by widespread adoption of eSource are so compelling as to ensure that the role of eSource will expand significantly. Increased adoption of eSource will lead to better quality, lower costs and higher productivity, just as the introduction of quality principles revolutionized the automobile industry.

CDISC-CW Survey

Sponsors and CROs almost unanimously agree that the application of data interchange standards is critical to the success of eClinical trial technology adoption. The vast majority of sponsors are either implementing or have plans to implement the data interchange standards developed through CDISC. According to the recent CDISC-CenterWatch survey, more than 90% of biopharmaceutical companies and CROs believe that data interchange standards should be extended to facilitate data collection at the investigative site level. Sponsors and CROs hope to reduce variability among data collection requirements and training needs across the wide variety of data systems used. The majority—89%—of investigative sites agree that sponsors should collaborate more actively in order to implement data interchange standards quickly and consistently. Biopharmaceutical and CRO companies also believe that the widespread implementation and adoption of data interchange standards will offer numerous benefits including decreased personnel time spent on data transfers, improved data quality and more efficient data exchange among partnering companies.

Facilitation of Site Processes

The first thing we can do to decrease work for the site is to cut the three to four data collection points to one or two. Sites already have the information on their patients' medical and medication histories needed for screening and enrollment of a trial subject. Why should coordinators have to re-enter all of this information onto a paper CRF just to have it re-entered into a database at the sponsor location? Or why should they re-enter it into an eCRF, which is an electronic representation of the paper case report form? Frequently, companies are so tied to the way they format paper CRFs that they insist on the exact representation on the screen, which makes it difficult to "think outside the box" and see how technology can vastly improve the current processes. With an eCRF (i.e., simply placing a case report form on a computer screen), the sponsor benefits from electronic data transfer, but the site personnel do not, because the work they do remains very much the same, but with somewhat easier centralized access and review.

If data could more readily be exchanged among systems, the following information could be collected once, not multiple times:

- Subject demographics and habits
- Medical history information
- Medication history
- Physical examinations
- Allergies or prior adverse events

Once a patient is enrolled into a clinical trial, data entered for the trial can generate the following information for the site:

- Patient visit status (pending data and/or outstanding queries)
- Protocol status and version of consent form
- Revenue recognition (based upon completed visits/procedures)
- Enrollment figures
- Patient management information, such as future visit scheduling
- Schedules for the coordinators, projecting patient visits

If a practice is already using electronic medical records, a recruitment database can be built using information in those records. Such site-based electronic medical records contain much of the initial data required for clinical trial recruitments. In addition, reports could be generated that show which patients are potential candidates for a trial, based upon inclusion/exclusion criteria. Many sites that conduct trials maintain separate recruitment databases and/or site management applications. Unfortunately, the data typically are not transferable from those applications into EDC applications. If such transfers were feasible, an investigator or coordinator could save a lot of time during the patient visit.

Other opportunities that could enhance efficiency for site personnel include direct capture of data from tools that measure ECGs or vital signs, automating IRB reports, or providing mechanisms to facilitate reporting of serious adverse events electronically. Sites could be compensated in a timely fashion based on the information that has been captured electronically and made available in real time to sponsors.

To turn these opportunities into reality and, more importantly, to conduct an optimal clinical trial, investigative sites must have the following needs met via process redesign leveraged with technology improvements.

- Reduced points of data collection and transcription/re-entry.
- Use of a cohesive system/processes for all trials vs. different ones for each trial and/or trial sponsor

- Standard interfaces, reducing the current need for coordinators and investigators to train on and learn numerous systems, sometimes simultaneously
- Site management tools that are integrated with data collection and interchange data with other tools and systems
- Integrated tools that enhance the site's processes with respect to conducting clinical trials while providing patient care, e.g., scheduling, patient contact information and trial information such as protocols and timelines
- Assurance that each of the possibly many computer systems and applications comply with FDA guidance and regulations
- Accelerated adoption of new technologies by the pharmaceutical industry

It is essential to keep site needs at the forefront of this process change because they are where collection of the initial data occurs. The site is the foundation of all of the subject data for clinical trials. Serving the sites facilitates more efficient collection of high quality data at the source, benefiting the industry as a whole.

Facilitation of Monitoring Processes

In addition to site personnel, CRAs or monitors have not always been accommodated adequately with new technologies to enhance their processes. Today, they must still physically go to the investigative sites to compare source documents with CRF data or eCRF data. When a CRA visits an investigative site, he or she has several objectives. The overall goal is to ensure that the trial is being conducted according to Good Clinical Practices. The CRA may check files for critical documents, ensure that drug storage is secure, ask if the site personnel have any questions or concerns and then spend the majority of their time ensuring that information in the medical record agrees with the paper CRFs and documenting when it is not. These issues/queries must then be addressed by the site before the data are transferred back to the sponsor.

If the CRF is placed online (eCRF) and the data are entered electronically, the monitor can review data before coming to the site and should receive cleaner data if edit checks are built in up front. The monitor can send queries to the site and have them resolved before a site visit. In addition, enrollment data can be tracked in real time so that the monitor can get a report indicative of the site's performance. This helps the monitor know whether a visit should be sooner or later than scheduled depending on how the site appears to be doing. Despite these benefits from new technologies, monitors still have to verify that the eCRF data are consistent with the paper source documents at the site.

Certain benefits for monitors already exist with EDC alone, such as reduced queries and possibly earlier and easier query resolution. Those benefits provide more accurate data earlier. However, areas remain that could be made easier by leveraging technology via an optimal clinical trial. Existing problems for monitors include the following:

- eSource data concepts are rarely implemented for more than the clinical lab data due to regulatory concerns and worries that sites initially may not be willing to enter data electronically.
- Many CRAs or monitors have "always done it that way" and thus have a difficult time transitioning to a new way of monitoring.
- A misperception persists that the monitor always has to double-check every entry because site personnel may be so busy that they make errors in the collection of the clinical trial data, or the physician may be too busy for a thorough review of data.
- Safety data are still often collected in applications other than the EDC tool, requiring cumbersome reconciliation steps. The advantages of technology in providing safety surveillance support is not yet adequately appreciated or utilized.
- Enhanced project/site management functionality has not been incorporated into many of the existing tools for EDC.
- Risk aversion or perceptions that sites and monitors will not use EDC tools, and continuing concerns about the regulatory expectations for monitoring electronic data capture during trials continue.
- Poorly developed EDC tools may require the monitor to do extra work just to use the system (e.g., too many clicks per page, slow or inadequate Internet connections, data synchronization issues).

Once again, existing technologies must be enhanced to deal with all the above issues adequately, and the industry needs to be willing to support all necessary and appropriate changes in existing processes.

> One EDC tool was designed such that, in order to change data after it had been reviewed internally, site personnel were required to call in to have the data unlocked to make the change. This was inconvenient for everyone involved. In response, site personnel started to add the new data to comment fields. It is a nightmare for a monitor or data manager to find information in comment fields that needs to be re-inserted into the proper field at a later date. By making the site process difficult for the sake of data monitoring and management, everyone suffered. It is important that the impact of any process change involving technology be evaluated across all users first.
>
> Note

Facilitation of Data Management Processes

Data management is an area where EDC tools have made a positive impact and have been developed with the users in mind. After all, many developers are in data management/biostatistics departments, or they are frequently contracted through these departments. Also, the data managers and statisticians understand data and the potential opportunities in managing clinical trial data appropriately.

The potential benefits of EDC for data management and other team personnel are:

- Reduction in data requiring clarification
- Facilitated query resolution
- Earlier access to data from sites
- Earlier indicators of site data entry problems or problems with data management programs
- More time to deal with real data management issues (e.g., getting systems up and running, and validation)
- Integrating data from multiple sources
- Managing the data on an ongoing basis such that the database lock can occur more quickly after the last data are available
- Facilitating awareness of data trends

Certain issues remain preventing data managers from reaping all of the potential benefits from electronic data capture. Some are the same as for the monitors, since these two groups are mainly responsible for ensuring the integrity and accuracy of the data. With the benefits of properly implemented technology, this locus of quality control can actually be shifted toward the point of origin at the site, where it has the greatest impact.

For data managers and others to realize the full potential of new technology for clinical trials, the following needs to happen:

- Sites need to be given the appropriate tools to minimize the transcription of data from source document to CRF worksheet to CRF.
- Safety data should be collected once, not again in a separate safety database, such that time-consuming reconciliation steps can be eliminated.
- The favorable regulatory expectations regarding electronic regulatory submissions and eClinical trial data must be made more widely known.
- There should be more focus on data fields or items (vs. forms/CRFs).
- Training needs to be provided and new skill sets encouraged within project teams to allow team members to become comfortable with new technologies.

Improved Communication and Coordination

Web-based technology applications offer important opportunities for improving clinical trials through enhanced global communications and coordination of processes for multi-center trials. New and relevant information can be distributed internationally in minutes, and issues can be raised to broad audiences or discretely, in real-time, as needed.

Project or educational information can be shared among distributed teams very effectively on the Internet. Some companies have found it to be a wonderful solution to managing SOPs and providing training. The Internet allows for team transactions to be readily shared in one place with one means. An optimal clinical trial would support all useful connectivity and communication among team members and preserve the record of such exchange to support "reconstruction" of the full context of the trial in the future under audit or regulatory review (see Chapter 7).

Improved Project Management

When communication and coordination among project team members improves, project management benefits. Again, new technologies, particularly web-based applications, provide many potential benefits for project managers, especially those with globally distributed project teams. Access to data in near real-time promotes earlier decisions and allows a manager to make changes as soon as possible when something is not going as planned (of course, no project goes completely as planned).

Project management is an area ripe to enjoy the benefits from new technologies applied to clinical trials. To manage the optimal clinical trial, these applications must address:

- Using available data (and ensuring a place for planned values prior to study start) to create project management views (e.g., planned vs. actual metrics). See Chapter 6, Metrics, for more information.
- Data interchange among different applications and external project management tools to eliminate redundant data entry.
- Ensuring that data are readily available in near real-time so that decisions can be made as soon as possible during a trial.
- Integrating project management information across different trials.
- The lack of an adequate baseline for metrics.
- The lack of appropriate metrics for making comparisons between paper-based trials and eCTs, e.g., many metrics used for paper-based trials are based on the number of CRF pages. ECT metrics should not be tied to CRFs; rather, they should focus on the more common factor of data fields.

Since certain companies tend to have far more data fields per CRF than other companies, having metrics based upon CRFs is actually not even an appropriate metric for paper-based trials.

Note

49

One interesting benefit for project managers for an eClinical trial is the requirement to plan adequately before study initiation. A paper-based process allows for the study to begin, patients to be enrolled and data to be collected before the database is built, even though that can negatively affect quality. A trial with electronic data collection, however, should not begin until the data collection tool, database, and data query system are all complete, validated and made accessible to the sites. In addition, metrics to be collected and the planned goals can and should be agreed upon ahead of time. While this has extended the planning time in some cases, this is every good project manager's ideal world—proper planning in advance.

Standardization

Chapter 10 deals further with industry standards for clinical data; however, it is worth mentioning both data standards and process standardization in the context of potential improvements for clinical trials. This is an important part of reaping the real value associated with conducting trials with new processes that leverage new technology. When process standards are created in one area, standardization can begin in other areas of the process. Each time one conducts a trial and uses what has been done in prior trials, the process is streamlined.

Sites collect much of the same data for every trial, such as subject demographics, medical history, pre-study (medication history) and concomitant medications, adverse events and end-of-study information. Many companies have designed certain standard case report forms. This way they can then standardize the database for these forms, edit checks for the standard data points, statistical analyses and so on. A domino effect is created. While standards can benefit certain processes, the domino effect can make the entire clinical trial more streamlined. Unfortunately, while different companies have developed standards for their processes, it can still translate to many ways of working for an individual investigative site or for a CRO. This makes it nearly impossible for sites or CROs to develop the standardized processes they need to be as efficient as possible. In an optimal clinical trial, such proprietary tools and attitudes will give way to standardization that will benefit the sites, CROs and other development partners, thus being beneficial for the biopharmaceutical companies in return.

This collaboration is actually happening with clinical data standards. The Clinical Data Interchange Standards Consortium (CDISC) consists of a growing group of clinical trials stakeholders, who are collaborating in the development of industry standards for data interchange. They began by developing standards for submission of data to regulatory authorities and then extending these to standards for electronically acquired data from various sources, including clinical lab data.

When developing such standards, it is best to look at the back end, or target, first. When data managers have some idea (of at least a core set) of the data that the FDA is going to want to review, these are clearly data that need to be collected, managed and analyzed. They may not encompass all of the data needed, since each protocol is different, but the core set is fairly well defined, particularly the safety data.

When one knows the data that are to be collected, the hypothesis and the objectives of the trial, the case report forms can be designed or, ideally, the data points that need to be collected can be identified independent of the forms. (This concept will also be important when metrics are discussed in Chapter 6.)

When data can be exchanged more readily among systems and technologies, then the opportunity of achieving a true eClinical trial starts becoming a reality. Numerous proprietary systems and applications would not be quite so cumbersome if there could be more commonality among the interfaces for the users, more standardization of the processes and a standard means of interchanging the data. Standards can also improve the quality and facilitate reviews. (For more about data standards, see Chapter 10.)

The Vision—Putting It All Together

We have now reviewed the goals of a true eClinical trial and concepts that could make this feasible. We have also addressed certain of the hurdles that still need to be addressed. One concept that has already been accepted in foreign countries and is not yet common in the United States is that of eSource documentation. The ultimate goal is to link the healthcare with clinical research and clinical trials in a way that patient safety is enhanced and clinical research is facilitated.

The vision of linking healthcare with clinical research is not a new one, but it has met widespread challenges. In order to achieve this, the following issues are either being addressed or must still be addressed:

- The regulatory requirements for clinical trial technology, as embodied by 21 CFR, Part 11, must be met by technology applied to healthcare environments.
- The patient privacy requirements of healthcare, as embodied by the Health Insurance Portability and Accountability Act (HIPAA), must be met by clinical research and the associated processes and tools.
- Physicians need to learn about and work toward being more accepting of technology such as electronic health records and electronic CRFs, and conversely these technologies should be developed to dovetail with physician workflow requirements, including those for clinical trials.
- Data interchange standards should address both healthcare and clinical trial data in a way that allows for secure interchanges of appropriate information.
- Pharmaceutical companies need to support sites by adopting and facilitating standard interfaces and processes for more efficient collection of high quality data at the site.

- Pharmaceutical companies need to embrace the concept of an optimal eCT and promote the standards and technology improvements needed to make these feasible.

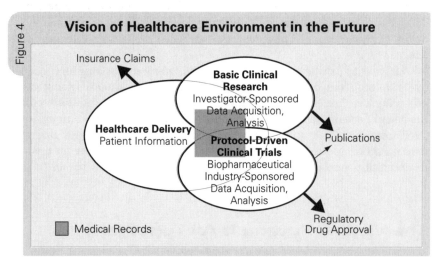

Figure 4

Vision of Healthcare Environment in the Future

There is a significant subset of information that could potentially be shared among the three areas that relate to healthcare: healthcare Delivery, Basic Clinical Research and Protocol-Driven Clinical Trials. The vision is such that such sharing would be mutually beneficial, in terms of time, effort and quality for improving patient care, not only among, but also within these areas.

In summary, table 1 compares certain features of trials conducted with paper processes, electronic data capture (EDC) and electronic clinical trials and an optimal eCT.

Table 1

	Paper	EDC	Optimal eCT
Electronic data collection	○	◗	●
Edit checks at entry point	○	◗	●
Primarily electronic processes	○	○	●
Integrated technology	○	◗	●
Built-in quality	○	◗	●
Facilitated monitoring	○	◗	●
Facilitated data management	○	◗	●
Improved comm./coord.	○	◗	●
Improved project management	○	◗	●
Standardization (data)	○	◗	●
Standardization (processes)	○	◗	●
Linked with healthcare	○	○	●

○ Not Available　◗ Variable Availability　● Available

Conclusion

Establishing the vision and setting the goals for an optimal electronic clinical trial are major steps in the effort toward achieving one. Many in the clinical industry may consider taking the time to look at how their processes work (or don't work) to be a step backward. The irony is that in order to move forward in achieving the goals of an electronic clinical trial, stakeholders will have to take a step back first to thoroughly study the various points in a study where errors and miscommunication occur. They will have to reduce the number of these points as well as improve communications among all parties involved in the conduct of the clinical trial. Such improvements can then lead to streamlined, redesigned processes better able to leverage technology and adopt standards.

Leveraging technology can also help streamline processes, but not if it is just another layer that is added on top of a process that is already sub-par. Technology is not the total solution, as we will see in the next chapter. The processes themselves must undergo change before technology can be implemented successfully. Then the technology requirements can be established and applications evaluated more appropriately.

Process Redesign and Supporting Technologies

Objectives

- Understand how clinical trial processes can be viewed with an eye toward improvement.
- List four steps that should be included in any process redesign.
- Describe four supporting technologies for clinical trials.
- List advantages and issues associated with these emerging technology solutions.

Introduction

In Chapter 3, we discussed the goals and benefits of an optimal eClinical trial (eCT). This chapter will describe the coupling of process redesign with supporting technology that must be achieved in order to conduct effective eCTs. Today, we have a host of new hardware, software and system offerings to support clinical trial conduct and complement process redesign. Most of these offerings are a result of new centralized software applications, infrastructure improvements in the areas of communications—broadband, wireless and Internet—or new hardware devices such as Personal Digital Assistants (PDAs) and tablet computers. These new technologies provide a basis for improvements in clinical trial conduct. They offer the opportunity for increased sharing of clinical data and trial information and, when coupled with redesigned processes, can facilitate the move toward an eCT environment.

Shredding the Paper—Process Redesign

If the conduct of clinical trials is going to improve and benefit from technology, clinical researchers must be willing to entertain the idea of adopting new processes with respect to emerging technology and reconsider the ways they have become accustomed to working. Researchers now know that they must improve on the current process of three-part NCR data collection forms (CRFs) placed in a binder on the shelf of a clinical research site, but the move to electronic clinical trials has been neither quick nor easy. Unfortunately, many of the first electronic data capture tools were conceived as point solutions and were frequently developed without sufficient consideration of the overall process. For this reason, many of the paper-based processes have been retained, and there has been a tendency simply to make a CRF into an eCRF. The result has been a marginal benefit at best.

> The initial name given to electronic data capture, remote data entry, is an interesting testimonial to early design considerations. RDE implies that the site is the remote location. In other words, RDE is a data management, or sponsor-centric, view of the clinical trials world. In practice, the site is the location where the data are conceived, and the sponsor is really the remote location. The term EDC is more appropriate as it does not represent such a sponsor-centric view.

Note

When an activity, such as a clinical trial, has been performed a certain way for so long, it is often hard even to begin thinking of ways to change and improve upon it. As an aid to getting started, consider the following steps:

1. Check assumptions and existing standard operating procedures (SOPs).
2. Map existing processes and potential new processes.
3. Compare processes and look for areas of improvement and/or elimination of steps.
4. Modify SOPs, if necessary, making certain to maintain compliance with regulations.

Check Assumptions

One good way to start clinical research process redesign is to list the facts or constraints the team is dealing with and then go through each one and question it. This is most effective when done as a group. Examples are often found in SOPs that are written for the way a company or organization has always done something, whereas the regulations do not necessarily have to be interpreted that way. SOPs are occasionally implemented as if they were regulations within a company, without thinking about their origins. It is wise to review the SOPs in the context of a new technology or process to ensure that the real meaning of the regulations is being implemented, and that compliance with regulations is maintained. The SOPs may then have to be modified.

Table 1

Fiction	Fact
Monitor visits should occur every 6 to 8 weeks (per SOP).	The monitor should visit the site frequently enough to ensure GCPs are being followed.
Monitoring data can only be done by visiting the site.	Data must accurately reflect source documentation.
Verifying the CRF back to source is the critical task.	The database must reflect the source documents.
The FDA will not accept eSource data.	eSource data are acceptable, albeit when meticulous attention is paid to systems technology validation and security. (Note: The FDA has been accepting eSource data for years in the form of clinical laboratory data.)
The CRF data fields drive the statistical analysis at the end of the trial.	The analysis and reviews that are intended to be done at the end of the trial should be defined in advance; therefore, the analysis plan drives the data fields.
To conduct a clinical trial, it is essential to have case report forms and that these be retained in paper form at the sites.	Electronic data are acceptable to the FDA providing that ALCOA considerations are followed, and the investigator maintains the data consistent with 21 CFR 12 (62.b). If data are collected electronically, they should be archived electronically.

Table 1 gives examples of certain fictions that have been thought of as fact, whereas often it is an existing SOP that has made them "factual." The actual facts from good clinical practices (GCPs) and other sources are listed in the fact column in this table. When considering supporting technologies, their implementation and effects on existing processes, be familiar with the relevant regulatory guidance documents and appropriate regulations. See Chapter 7 for relevant regulatory information. Also, be aware that guidance documents from regulatory agencies may be interpreted differently by different regulators. It is best to discuss specific systems and situations with the responsible regulators. (However, the move toward clinical data standards may reduce this need in the future.) Remember, guidance is just that—guidance—and does not hold the force of law as do regulations.

Map the Existing and New Processes

After evaluating SOPs for fact versus fiction, continue with process redesign by mapping out potential new process(es) and making a comparison with the existing or baseline processes. Process mapping can even be done before choosing supporting technology. Once mapped, if the new process does not make improvements, researchers must ask themselves why. Perhaps the way the technology is going to be applied is ineffective, or someone has not thought of a new, and better, way to do things.

Figures 1 and 2 are examples of two process maps—one for an existing paper-based clinical trial process and one for an eSource web-based clinical trial. The first process map is one that shows the steps for a paper-based trial, as was presented in Figure 1 in Chapter 2.

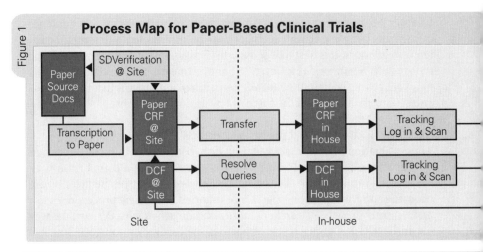

Process Map for Paper-Based Clinical Trials

Figure 1

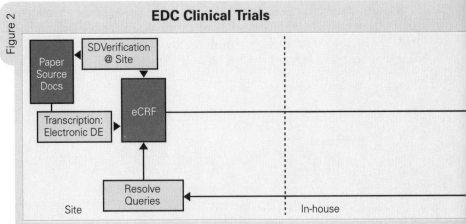

EDC Clinical Trials

Figure 2

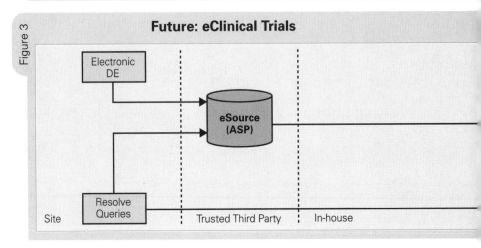

Future: eClinical Trials

Figure 3

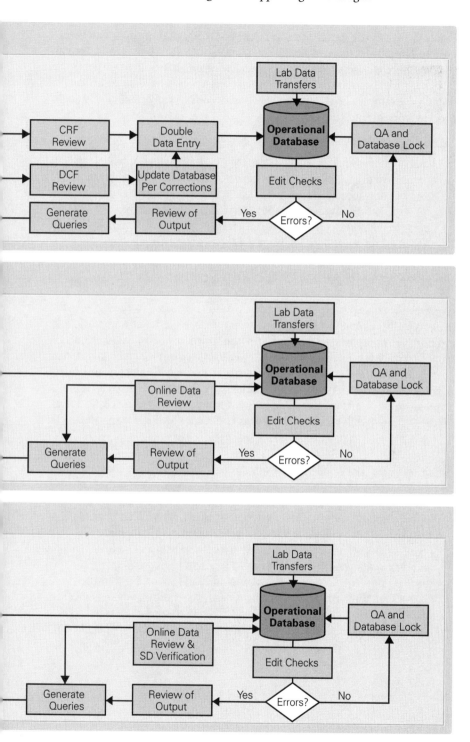

Compare Processes

Figure 2 reveals the simplification achieved by leveraging supporting technology. Not only is this simpler at first glance, but with a closer look one can see that there is access to information by far more parties at an earlier point in time. The elimination of steps and access to cleaner data at an earlier point are examples of the value that would not typically emerge if the old process were simply automated.

> **Note**
>
> A number of people have said that Figure 1 gives them a headache or makes them uncomfortable when looking at it! Who could blame them! Unfortunately, this is actually a kind version of the paper process used for the majority of trials today. And this one does not even include the use of a CRO. The complexity of Figure 1 should tell us something without even having to read each symbol in the flow chart.

It is essential to keep in mind that it is not necessary to re-engineer the process to this extent all at once. The technology, experience and regulatory environment may not yet be ready for the ultimate vision of an electronic clinical trial. Each integration of systems; each removal of redundant data entry and repetitive processes generates cost savings, timeliness and safety advantages if coupled with a re-engineered process and proper training. Some of the benefits are available today through an electronic clinical trial. Figure 3 shows what an eSource process could look like when mapped.

> **Note**
>
> One re-engineering team took a foam core board and put pins at each handoff for a CRF. Then, they strung white string between the pins. An amazing number of handoffs, more than 50, were discovered, for a CRF that went through two rounds of query resolution or data clarification between data management, monitoring, the study coordinator and others on the team. (Note that two rounds is certainly not atypical in a paper-based process.) However, when the team strung a colored string between handoffs for a CRF that had no queries, the path was significantly less treacherous. This colorful path should be the norm, if discrepancies are identified when and where they occur, rather than once the CRF is in-house.

Metrics for Assessing Newly Introduced Technology

While we discuss metrics in Chapter 6 in depth, it is appropriate here to illustrate how they can be used to assess a newly introduced technology. After creating a process map of the current process and the new process, it's easier to see in the new process where metrics pertain and how they apply when certain steps have been deleted. Then, one can best see where metrics can be compared across different processes. New technologies can also bring in additional metrics possibilities, such as system performance.

Following are examples of process maps that were developed with the intent of assessing the performance and benefits of an EDC (eCRF) system vs. a paper system (Figure 4), and an EDC (eCRF) system vs. an eClinical trial process that includes eSource (Figure 5). An appropriate assessment of a new system may also include subjective evaluations, such as what different users, e.g., the site personnel and the CRAs, think about a system.

For Figures 4 and 5, metrics that can be collected and compared include:

1 = Time to set up system (elapsed time from final protocol available to first site initiated) reported as hours, if possible.
2 = Time to document source data into patient record (specific visit and/or cycle).
3 = Time to enter data into eCRF (specific visit and specific page(s) and elapsed time from source documentation).
4 = Time to monitor (per site, per patient), including time for data review and clarification in-house and at-site + travel.
5 = Time (average) to resolve a query and number of queries through a specific visit/cycle, by patient and by data field.
6 = Time to finalize data for a certain visit and/or cycle per patient.

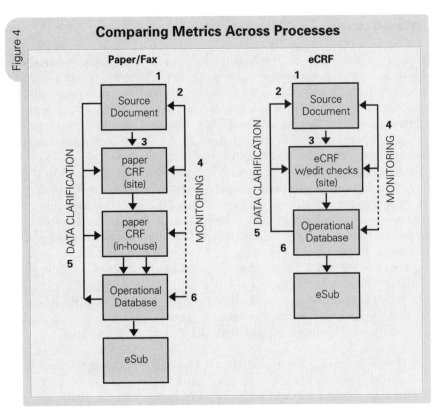

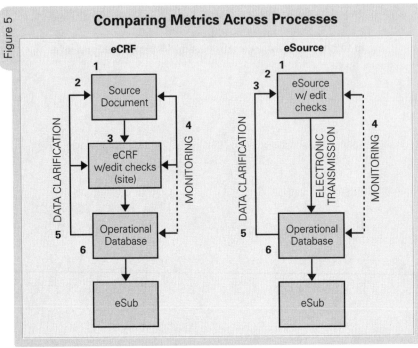

Supporting Technologies and Services for eCTs

Despite the opportunities and benefits that various supporting technologies and new applications can provide, particularly when combined with a redesigned clinical trial process, the clinical trials industry has yet to fully benefit from the majority of these. Today, it is estimated that 90% or more of trials conducted still rely on the paper-based process with three-part NCR data collection forms (CRFs) placed in a binder (casebook), despite the fact that the FDA encourages the use of properly designed electronic systems in clinical trials and electronic NDA submissions.

The following sections will provide overviews of several of the most promising technologies—the Internet, Application Service Provider model, handheld devices, broadband, wireless.

Internet

Most uses of the Internet for clinical trials to date have focused on EDC. Earlier, we presented additional areas of clinical trials where efficiencies and accuracies can be obtained through coordination, collaboration and centralization using the Internet. As the Internet becomes more widely applied to clinical trials, processes such as randomization, medication dispensing, monitoring, AE reporting, site financial reimbursement and sponsor reports can be conducted much more efficiently. Its use for data collection will also grow.

Key advantages of the Internet are the dissemination of clinical trial information and the coordination of multiple clinical trial processes. Web portals can provide readily comprehensible views of the data in different forms and from different applications. Web-based visualization tools can facilitate assimilation of relevant information quickly to see where the drill-down for more details needs to occur. These tools and views can also accommodate a number of protocols concurrently.

> Some readers will remember the days when personal financial transactions were conducted by paper; checks took days or weeks to process. The delay in processing was referred to as "float," and it generally was undesirable and represented inefficiencies in the system. The application of computer systems to the banking industry dramatically reduced the float, in some cases to seconds. Clinical trials have "information float"—the time delay in making trial data available to those team members who need access to the data. Minimizing information float is a reasonable and realizable goal.
>
> Note

Using the Internet for EDC and the clinical trial processes identified here will lead to gains in efficiencies and accuracy of study conduct while also better meeting FDA requirements for valid audited study data.

One of the principal ways that Internet applications will be used in clinical trials is via Application Service Providers, often in conjunction with a Trusted Third Party (TTP). In fact, one of the greatest potential advantages of the ASP model is its ability to address regulatory, privacy and security issues when used in conjunction with a trusted third party. Maintaining data integrity is essential to the success of electronic systems in clinical trials. Information technology (IT) has many tools to achieve data integrity. However, without proper attention to software and systems, it is possible to compromise the verifiable integrity of data in a clinical trial. In an online system with a TTP, the investigator may not retain a copy of the eCRF or eSource at the site during the trial. If paper source is retained at the site, it is imperative that the paper source match or be reconciled with the data stored at the TTP.

The concept of a TTP for the conduct of electronic clinical trials is a very useful tool to address regulatory issues. The TTP could be a technology vendor capable of authenticating transactions and also hosting and managing the database for the clinical trial. A key requirement, though, is that access to those data remains under the control of the investigator throughout the trial. The sponsor, however, can arrange for data transfers or to obtain data "streams" at appropriate time intervals during the course of the trial. The TTP must have SOPs and procedures in place that assure that data are not improperly manipulated or changed. The use of the TTP provides additional assurance that the integrity of the trial data has not been compromised.

Application Service Provider (ASP) Models

In the application service provider (ASP) model, applications reside on a server located at the ASP and are either distributed to sites via a network or used centrally through a web browser. The sites access the software over the Internet or a private network and use the application as needed. If executed properly, the user is not aware that the application is running remotely, and the user has continuous, real-time access to the application. Neither the software nor any data remain on the local PC. All application functionality is delivered over the network to site computers, and all data generated during a session is stored on the ASP servers.

This model is a major change from commonly used software distribution models that involve distribution of software via some physical medium such as a CD-ROM. Since the applications can be hosted and supported remotely in the ASP model, customers do not need an extensive Information Technology (IT) group to support these applications. In an ideal world, it provides a means to level the playing field between smaller customers and larger customers.

Some clinical trial ASP applications require the transfer of large amounts of application data; in this case, reliable, affordable, persistent, high-bandwidth connectivity between data entry sites and a host computer is essential. Even if the applications do not require large amounts of data, it is desirable to have the high-bandwidth connectivity in order to give the end user better performance.

The ASP approach can produce a centralized information and management environment in which authorized users can have greater insight into the operation of the clinical trial. When implemented properly, the site has control of and access to their own data. The sponsor can monitor in real-time a specific site's activity during the trial and have more information about study conduct across all sites at an earlier point in time. Clinical data are stored in a single central database; consequently, this approach can offer more security since data are not stored at a large number of distributed sites. The investigative site does not have to develop a specific trial infrastructure to support an ASP application. The ASP model offers the potential for significant changes in the conduct of a clinical trial.

The ASP model offers more control of trial processes than does the decentralized model, allowing checking of data elements against predetermined ranges and comparing data elements across sites during study conduct. The ASP model makes study data available in near real-time for monitoring and checking, resulting in earlier and ongoing data cleaning. This, in turn, facilitates an earlier database lock.

In summary, the ASP model offers the following potential advantages:

- **Reduced Local Software Maintenance.** With the ASP model, everyone has the potential to access the same software and data at the same time, thus eliminating the need to maintain separate copies, installations and customizations of the software and to reconcile data across databases.
- **Enhanced Information Sharing.** As long as a user has a suitable network connection and the necessary security clearance, he or she can access clinical trial information, so sharing information becomes much easier.
- **Ease of Upgrades.** Software upgrades can be applied readily, as appropriate.
- **Robust Crash Protection.** If a site computer crashes, any data that have been transferred remain safe on the ASP server. This reduces the time and money spent on proprietary systems and allows more time and money to be spent on the actual work of the clinical trial. Software and data backup issues are the responsibility of the ASP.
- **Reduced Staff Cost.** The convenience features of ASPs take a great burden off of the site IT staff.
- **Trusted Third-Party Provision.** The ASP model can offer a provision to have a trusted third party, i.e., a neutral party, that hosts the data for both site and sponsor and provides security and authentication services. The differing needs for data access and certain issues of subject confidentiality can be accommodated through such a neutral mechanism, whereas hosting the database at the sponsor site precludes the inclusion of certain information the site may want to maintain access.

However, the ASP model also raises the following potential issues:

- **Longevity.** Numerous ASPs organizations have attempted to enter the market, and many have disappeared. It is essential to work with ASPs that have a proven track record and financial stability.
- **Back-up.** Since clinical data (in some cases, eSource) resides on the ASP computers, it is essential that procedures are in place at the ASP to guarantee no loss of data.
- **Performance.** It must be verified that the user requirements in terms of response and availability are met.

Handheld Devices

Small handheld devices, such as offline and wireless palm devices, are being used increasingly in clinical trials. These devices are often appropriate for collecting direct subject information such as diary information. Rather than collect information in paper diaries to be returned at a later date to the physician, diary information can be collected and stored in a handheld device and subsequently transferred electronically for storage in the study database. Since the functionality of these devices continues to expand, they might serve a larger role in the future. Models are becoming available that combine PDA functionality with cell phone capability; this opens up the possibility of real-time data collection and enhanced interactivity between study participants and site personnel. For example, it would be possible for the cell phone capability to be used to remind subjects to enter data. Tablet computers and logpads are also beginning to be used in clinical settings. A tablet computer more closely approximates the conventional patient chart and offers the advantage that the data are directly entered in electronic format.

However, the use of handheld or tablet devices to store source data places additional constraints on the management of these devices. If the handheld device is lost or stolen before source data can be transferred to a more persistent storage medium, then the site runs the risk of losing irreplaceable data and violating patient confidentiality guidelines. The marriage of handheld and tablet devices with wireless technology at a site could result in more system infrastructure at the site and more points of failure. It also introduces additional security considerations. Although most wireless healthcare applications come with some security features, existing safeguards are not foolproof. An industry-wide wireless standard to protect the transfer of sensitive data does not yet exist. At this point in time, users will need to evaluate each wireless system to validate that the system offers adequate security measures. The use of cell phone capability eliminates the site infrastructure issues, but does not necessarily solve the security issues.

As PDAs, tablet computers and logpads become more widely used and the technology matures, these may form a viable option for collecting data in real time during the subject's visit, rather than entering data on paper and then transcribing it later into a computer. PDAs and cell phones are now being used in numerous trials for which patients provide certain data themselves.

Broadband

As clinical trial applications mature, there will be a greater demand for the transfer of increasing amounts of data such as radiology images, ECG waveform data and other clinical data. The transfer of such image data requires broadband connectivity. In addition, even clinical trial applications that are designed to work effectively on dial-up connections are substantially enhanced when used over broadband connections.

Broadband is typically taken to mean data rates of at least 128 kilobits/second (typical dial-up modem connections are 3 to 40 kilobits/second). Large organizations have the opportunity to distribute the cost of broadband connectivity to their many users through T1 (or higher), fiber optic, microwave, laser and satellite links. Today, it is becoming realistic for small organizations and even individual users to achieve broadband access to the Internet through Digital Subscriber Lines (DSL) or cable modems. An advantage of DSL is that it operates over existing phone lines, so connectivity is already in place but a disadvantage is that it can typically only be offered in locations within approximately four miles of a central telephone office. Various techniques are emerging to expand the reach of DSL, but the use of existing cabling will always place limits on the data rates that can be achieved. Cable access may be more advantageous than DSL, if it is available in the local area of an investigative site and if the cable operator has provided adequate infrastructure. Unlike DSL, cable access is usually shared among many users, so it is important that the cable provider provide the segmentation necessary for adequate performance. Satellite-based, Internet broadband connectivity for individuals and small business is a much smaller market segment than either DSL or cable and has some unique issues when applied to eClinical trials. The advantage of satellite is that it is available to just about anyone (in the Northern Hemisphere) who can mount a dish antenna capable of seeing the southern sky. However, satellite is typically more expensive than DSL or cable, performance can be affected by weather conditions and it is subject to significant (typically 0.5 second to 0.75 second) time delays for each transaction.

Cable, DSL and bidirectional satellite connections are all capable of inbound (e.g., to the site) data transfer rates of approximately a megabit per second; transfer rates from the site are typically lower and range from hundreds of kilobits per second up to megabits per second. The most commonly offered DSL is called ADSL or asymmetric DSL. The modems are configured to achieve the highest rate on the inbound data transfer. For additional cost, a subscriber can often purchase symmetric DSL (SDSL) to get equal inbound and outbound data rates. Investigative sites with broadband access to the Internet will have a distinct advantage in competing for and participating in clinical trials in the future, as site efficiency should be significantly enhanced through the enhanced communication capabilities.

One caveat for any user interested in broadband connectivity is to evaluate vendors carefully before subscribing. Check references with special attention to performance and service. Also confirm that the vendor is financially stable; there has been extensive vendor fallout, especially among the DSL providers.

Since these broadband connections provide continuous connectivity, it is essential that a site take appropriate measures to safeguard computers and network. This is always the best practice for computer security. Software and hardware solutions are readily available. The demand for such devices has reduced firewall protection to near commodity status. Cost and performance of most hardware-based devices does not vary greatly; however, the ease of set-up and maintenance should be considered carefully before finalizing a purchase. Security measures should also include automated protection against viruses and the ability to continuously update the virus protection.

Wireless

Using the Internet for clinical trials conduct requires a network connection of sufficient speed for information transfer between the host computer and local PC. A disadvantage of wired systems is that the PC or PDA is constrained to the location where the connection exists. Wireless connectivity links a PC or PDA to a central computer. There are two basic types of wireless connections that are analogous to wireless telephone service. The first is a wireless Local Area Network (LAN), which is analogous to a cordless home telephone. A wireless LAN is very inexpensive to install (less than $500 for a small office system), has no ongoing costs associated with it and transmits high (11-50 mbit/sec) bandwidth information over relatively short ranges. It is perfect for sharing broadband Internet connection between local computers in a physician's practice. It is easily achievable today and is reasonably (but not completely) secure as long as encryption is used. Wireless LANs are used instead of wiring in many homes and offices today.

The second type of wireless connection is the wireless Wide Area Network (WAN), in which a mobile computer has direct wireless Internet connection. The wireless WAN is very similar to a cell phone—it requires towers at regular intervals, is very spotty in coverage in the U.S. at the time of this printing, has monthly charges, and has not yet achieved high bandwidth connectivity. The typical bandwidth of a wireless WAN is similar to the bandwidth of a dial-up connection. While this is bound to improve, wireless WANs are best used today for very low bandwidth communications—the transfer of emails in special pagers or the viewing of simple web pages.

Security is a major issue with wireless networks. It's very easy to eavesdrop without detection on the wireless traffic, so all clinical data must be adequately encrypted.

Conclusion

To make the improvements necessary for electronic clinical trials, the changes may seem at first to be a bit difficult since the technology to be leveraged is quite new. However, it is quite clear that advances in areas such as the Internet, ASP product delivery, handheld devices, broadband and wireless can enable significant improvements in the way trials are conducted, particularly with respect to the acquisition and distribution of the electronic data. In addition, these advances will open up an entire spectrum of opportunities for improving the complete process of bringing project teams together and new drugs and devices to market. It will be possible to provide near real-time data to team members; the quality of the data will improve and the ease of working with the data will be enhanced. In principle, most of the transactions should become electronic, rather than stay paper-based.

Although an eCT offers significant advantages to all the stakeholders in the clinical trial, this is not sufficient to guarantee acceptance by everyone. In order to partake of these advantages, the paper-based process must be redesigned, not just made electronic with new technology. People will have to change the way they work. Human nature does not always accommodate the seamless acceptance of this change—even if the change is beneficial. The implication is that the introduction of the new processes and technology must be carefully planned in conjunction with those involved. Involvement by all the affected parties before critical decisions are made is preferable to presenting the results and expecting the results to be embraced. Additional considerations with respect to resourcing project teams for eCT are covered in the following chapter.

IMPLEMENTATION

CHAPTER

Achieving eClinical Trials

Objectives

- List five basic elements to address for implementation with respect to achieving eClinical Trials.
- Be able to list essential evaluation criteria for selecting vendors and/or new technologies for clinical trials.
- List five special considerations to explore when planning an electronic clinical trial.

Introduction

Although we cannot yet realistically expect that every trial will be an "optimal" trial, we need to maintain that vision and strive to achieve it, if we are ever to get there. We know that not only are we faced with the challenge of redesigning our processes in a way that will leverage technology, but we must also select from many potential options for new technologies. Most pharmaceutical companies have started slowly with respect to implementing new clinical trials technology, and for the most part they have only seen incremental improvements. Few have already begun changing their entire organization to support eClinical trials (eCTs), although many have corporate goals to do this over the course of the next few years. Since clinical trials are costly and lengthy endeavors, we cannot afford to have them fail due to processes or technology. All too often they fail for other reasons. So, what is a realistic expectation, especially in the initial eCTs? How do we take the leap of faith that is necessary to reap the most benefits an eCT has to offer? How can we be made comfortable with the associated risks?

This chapter provides certain basic elements and selection criteria to assist in the implementation stages for eCTs. There are, of course, different versions of these steps and criteria that may work best for different organizations. Reaching a corporate goal requires organizational change with top-level management support and communication. New technology and processes applied to a trial by a project team constitutes important progress toward such a goal. But they do not address the overall organizational and industry issues, which should be kept in mind as part of the ultimate vision.

Elements for Implementing eClinical Trials

We have discussed that the processes involved when utilizing new and supporting technologies are very important. When discussing implementation for an eClinical Trial, we must begin by addressing certain critical factors or elements that must be incorporated from the beginning.

PRISM

One approach to planning eClinical Trials can be distilled under the acronym PRISM: planning, resourcing, implementation, support and management/metrics. These basic elements are not all that different from those required for paper trials. However, proper consideration must be given in advance to the process redesign, the selection of technology and the anticipated changes from the standard process in order that the implementation steps can result in an improvement over the paper-based clinical trial process.

P Planning

R Resourcing

I Implementation

S Support

M Management/Metrics

Planning

The PRISM process, first and foremost, emphasizes the Planning stage, which is where quality is built in from the beginning, as we discussed in

Chapter 3. Proper and complete planning upstream minimizes costly errors and significantly decreases rework downstream. Planning is a critical time when introducing a new technology or new processes. All too often it gets short shrift in favor of getting the trial started.

Planning not only includes project-specific planning but it begins with the process redesign steps. Once these steps have been completed, per the prior chapter, the new process can be put into play. It is highly recommended that a master plan be developed at the beginning of every trial; some have called this a MAP (Master Action Plan). Actually, one can develop a template that can be used repeatedly and then simply customized when a specific trial is being planned so that nothing is forgotten. Not only does a MAP serve as a team planning and communication tool during the planning stages, it should be a "living document" that is modified as needed during the trial. With new web-based applications, this plan can be posted on the web for all team members to access as needed.

Planning for an electronic clinical trial should at minimum address the following:

- Protocol design and designation of key safety and efficacy criteria/endpoints
- Statistical analysis plan
- Identification of data points to be collected
- Project team resourcing
- Standardization (industry standards and other applicable standards)
- Evaluation of new technology to be employed
- Processes, including use of new technology (overall steps and process maps)
- Master Trial Implementation Plan
  - Timelines
  - Goals and metrics
  - Communication methods
  - Requirements specification (see Chapter 7)
  - Technology (e.g., process implications, trial-specific customization needs, validation, roll-out, support)
  - Data quality measures
  - Data management plan (e.g., edit checks, data verification, security, archive, retention)
  - Site selection criteria
  - Training (site personnel and project team members)
  - Subject recruitment strategy
  - Regulatory compliance considerations
  - IRB submission and approval process
  - Clinical laboratory specification
  - Safety monitoring plan and adverse event reporting
  - Change control
  - Risk management procedures

It may appear at first glance that there are too many items under Planning. However, as a colleague phrased it: "People don't plan to fail; they fail to plan." Planning is crucial to a good outcome.

Electronic clinical trials require that many steps that frequently take place in the paper world after the trial has begun must take place before the trial begins. In a comparison across trials, we have found that a well-written MAP that included a detailed data management plan that was well communicated to the team in advance reduced incoming errors well over fifty-fold. This was true even for trials that did not use new technology for data collection.

Master plan templates can facilitate the planning stages such that adding the new technology does not become a rate-limiting factor. For example, master plans that provide for: establishing adequate infrastructure (networks, connectivity, security) at the sites; training of personnel in selected areas (e.g., regulatory issues that affect the use of computers in clinical trials) associated with eCTs; and training on the new applications being used for the trial. As eCTs become more prevalent, the type and amount of support will decrease, but it's essential now that these items be carefully considered during the planning stage.

Resourcing

People are critical to the success of the process, particularly when using a new technology. When a team member is unwilling to try new tasks, it may have a negative impact on other team members. This could, in turn, compromise the outcome of the trial. eClinical Trials should remove tasks that are associated with paper-based processes. Some view this as a positive step, and others may feel it is a threat to their position. At the same time, different tasks or challenges may arise, which may elicit varying responses or require role changes for individuals on an eCT project team.

It is also important to provide training to the project team (which includes site personnel), particularly on the new technology that is to be used for eCTs. One objective of training on a new technology is to elicit and strengthen buy-in by the users. If the project team members are flexible, want to learn and excel, and find new challenges interesting and exciting, the chances of success are higher.

Implementation

The Implementation stage is a matter of putting the planning into action, monitoring the progress and then identifying and making necessary modifications as soon as possible. There is actually not much more that needs to be addressed with respect to this stage. If the plan is a good one and is executed by capable individuals, then the chances of success are very good. The other elements that are important to a successful implementation stage are that there is adequate support for the technology and that the management procedures (and metrics to monitor the progress) have been built into the planning stage.

Support

Support is critical to a team implementing a technology-enabled project. Both clinical and technical support must be available around the clock to take care of the unexpected and the routine questions that arise. When a technology application is well designed and appropriate training is provided, the questions about how to use the tool are minimal and then decrease significantly as user experience increases; however, having help available when it is needed is very important to the users.

Management/Metrics

Management activities are facilitated via real-time, online information and metrics with which to gauge performance, thus driving informed decisions to the earliest point. The use of metrics for eClinical Trials is addressed in the Chapter 6. It is important to reach agreement in advance within the project team on primary objectives of the clinical trial and the implementation of new processes and technology. It is also important to consider the objectives from a corporate perspective. Subject safety, compliance with regulations and quality should always be among the primary objectives for eCTs; the relative importance of other objectives needs to be agreed upon up front. For example, is it important to lock a database quickly or to have access to cleaner data sooner than with the existing process? Or, is the primary objective staying on budget for the trial? Once the primary objectives are established, the metrics can be designated and means to monitor them on an ongoing basis can be addressed.

Facilitating project management via eClinical Trials is one of the key goals for an optimal trial. At this point, it makes sense to address the criteria that can be used to evaluate and select technology that will facilitate this move to eClinical Trials.

Technology and Vendor Selection Criteria

Each company will need to develop its own list of technology and vendor selection criteria, based upon its priorities. However, there is a core list of requirements, such as regulatory compliance and user acceptance of technology, that all companies should include. (A traceability matrix, which traces how software products comply with 21 CFR, Part 11 regulations can be found in Appendix D.) An initial list of issues that should be addressed in terms of identifying the requirements follows.

Important overall considerations in selecting new technology solutions include:

- Ensuring that the new technology will indeed facilitate the new processes and that the processes will leverage the technology.
- Ensuring that the technology will "grow" with the changing environment and not become obsolete in a very short period of time.

- Ensuring that the technology supports data interchange standards such that the data can be shared with minimal re-entry or cumbersome integration procedures.

Vendor and Product Evaluation Criteria

Table 1

Evaluation Criteria	Issue
Vendor Background	Clinical trial experience
	Software development experience
	Commitment to area
	International experience
	Financial stability
	References
Product Specifications	
— Regulatory and Standards	Security
	Compliance with 21 CFR 11
	Compliance with ICH GCP guidelines
	Compliance with HIPAA
	Conformance with FDA Guidance: Computerized Systems Used in Clinical Trials
	Compliance with CDISC standards
— User	Ease of use
	Performance
	Query resolution
	Data viewing
	Management tools
	Reports
	Data export and import
	Specific user requirements, e.g., compatibility with existing systems, low bandwidth connectivity
	Other value-added features
— Operational	Ease of setup
	Technical support
	Support for international studies
	Training
	Ease of upgrades and enhancements
	Need for customization
— Business	Pricing
	Contract terms
	Service level agreements

Special Implementation Considerations for eCTs

Following the key elements for achieving electronic clinical trials and using the essential criteria for assessing new technologies should be helpful to any project team that wants to achieve a successful eCT. There are, however, certain special implementation issues that deserve more consideration than can be given in one chapter. While these generally apply to any clinical trial, they deserve additional attention when conducting an eCT. These implementation issues are listed below, and each has one of the following chapters dedicated to it.

- **Metrics for Electronic Clinical Trials.** There is no reason to conduct an eCT if it does not improve upon today's clinical trial. Objective metrics are necessary to establish where the benefits are reaped and also to know where improvements can still be made. Because many of the metrics used for today's trial do not necessarily apply to eCTs (e.g., CRF flow), careful consideration of how success will be measured in the planning stage of an eCT is warranted. Chapter 6 explores the use of metrics for eCTs.

- **Performing Electronic Clinical Trials in Accord with the Regulations.** There are certain regulations, such as 21 CFR, Part 11, and regulatory guidance documents that apply specifically to eCTs. These regulations and guidance documents may be difficult to readily interpret, in terms of how they apply to a new technology. In addition, the guidance documents are just that, guidance. They are to be used as guides and do not have the force of law. Regulators are open to discussing how a company interprets 21 CFR, Part 11 and its guidance documents, provided the company can justify its interpretation based on the regulatory language. Chapter 7 discusses regulations that are relevant to eCTs.

- **Data Quality and Data Integrity.** Chapter 8 provides an exploration of data quality and data integrity in a clinical trial. It covers error sources and discusses steps that can be taken to improve the probability of capturing data that are accurate, consistent and reflect a patient's experience in a clinical study. It also emphasizes the importance of generating a data quality plan that includes reasonable metrics for data quality.

- **The Impact of eCT on Safety Surveillance and IRBs.** Chapter 9 focuses on safety surveillance and IRBs and the way that eCTs have an impact on these areas of clinical trials. The roles and responsibilities of the investigator, the medical monitor, the FDA and IRBs associated with an electronic clinical trial are outlined. The issue of patient privacy and its relationship to eCTs are also covered in detail.

- **Industry Standards for Electronic Clinical Data Interchange.** Because of the numerous choices available for new technologies and the fact that these are primarily point solutions, it is important to ensure that the data collected will transfer between systems readily, without tedious mapping and integration procedures. The progress in the area of clinical data interchange standards now makes it feasible to plan for ready data interchange among multiple organizations and technologies. Chapter 10 provides information that is essential to consider when selecting technology and streamlining the eCT process overall.

Conclusion

Achieving successful eCTs is much like achieving any successful clinical trial. However, there are certain distinct differences that are important to recognize in the planning stage. In this chapter, we explored the concept of PRISM in terms of key steps to follow, and a table providing basic criteria to assist in the evaluation and selection of a new technology was presented. We also provided an overview of implementation issues that are unique to eCTs.

While we must be realistic about what we can expect to achieve today, companies should nevertheless set their sights high. If the industry is going to move from paper or EDC to conducting repeatable, optimal eCTs, it must move from automating the existing processes and conducting pilot studies with new technology to the actualization of the goals that were presented in Chapter 3. This means that a new technology must address more than the standard checklist of criteria for evaluation; it must also support the vision, as described in that chapter.

Recall that, if the industry is to redesign and simplify the current clinical trials processes and improve them dramatically by leveraging technology, several goals, as described in Chapter 3, should be reached. These goals include: built-in quality, facilitation of site processes, facilitation of monitoring processes, facilitation of data management processes, improved communication and coordination, improved project management and standardization.

The next five chapters explore in more depth special implementation considerations, including metrics, regulations, data quality and integrity, patient safety and data interchange standards. All of these considerations provide information that is useful in conducting a successful eCT.

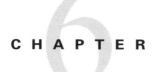

CHAPTER

Measuring and Managing for Success: Metrics for Electronic Clinical Trials

Objectives

- Understand what metrics are and why they are useful in clinical trials.
- List metrics that are useful as indicators of clinical trial performance and identify key metrics.
- Compare metrics appropriate for eClinical trials with those typically tracked for paper-based trials.

Introduction

New technologies and the Internet provide an opportunity for the industry to take a leap forward. Through the leveraging of technology to improve their processes, the clinical trials industry will join other industries that reaped increases in efficiencies. But how can trial managers and sponsors determine whether they are reaping the expected benefits and meeting their goals? And, how can clinical research professionals know the status of a clinical trial and whether it is going well or there is a problem that should be addressed? If properly collected and used, metrics can help us answer these questions.

Metrics are forms of measurement. Studies on quality and continuous process improvement have shown that measuring indicators of performance and making these known to those involved improves performance.

This makes sense, but unfortunately it is not always easy to determine what should be measured. Having determined what is to be measured, it can be difficult to obtain the measurements, report them and then use them for making decisions on process and quality improvement in a timely manner.

If collected and used appropriately, metrics should not only indicate where improvement is needed but also where there are areas of success. They should not only facilitate and encourage continuous improvement but also:

- Act as a management or decision-making tool.
- Enable benchmarking with others in the industry. (The ability to benchmark is a reason to standardize metrics and the associated definitions across the industry.)
- Increase effective communication throughout the organization by providing objective information and reducing opportunities for ambiguity.
- Provide opportunities for early problem identification and correction.
- Permit the consistent tracking of identified project objectives.

Clinical Trials Metrics Collection

Certain metrics are tracked for most clinical trials. These are typically cycle time metrics—measurements of time between one milestone and another. The most frequent metric cited for clinical trials is the time between when the last subject enrolled completes the last visit to when the database is considered clean enough to be "locked." It is at that point that the blind can be broken and the results analyzed. This is an important metric because this period of time is considered non-value-added. Shortening this time period is important to those conducting the clinical trial because during this time researchers cannot know the results of a blinded trial. Fortunately, this cycle time is also relatively easy to measure. In addition to the cycle time from last subject complete to database lock, other commonly tracked cycle time metrics include: time from protocol approved to first subject enrolled; time from first subject enrolled to last subject enrolled; and time from database lock to report complete. In fact, these have become fairly standard metrics in the clinical trials industry, perhaps because benchmarking companies have made an effort to compare these across clinical trials and across companies, and in doing so they have created certain *de facto* metrics, at least for the comparative work.

Defining Terms Used in Common Metrics

Terms used in common metrics must be defined in advance. For example, when defining the milestone, database lock, there are several related terms that different companies use, depending upon their processes and their standard operating procedures. There could be a process that includes a database "close" or a "soft lock," which is followed by a quality assurance assessment to determine the error rate of the database. After this the database is locked if the error rate is acceptable, or the data are cleaned more if the error rate is unacceptable. Another company may not use the terms "close" or "soft lock." In other processes, a company may allow the unlocking of the database. For example, if issues are found during the analysis process, they will allow it to be unlocked to make a change in the data and then locked again, as long as there is appropriate documentation on what was changed and the required signatures to verify that this was properly done. Still another company may lock the database only once and never allow an unlock, but continue to document problems it finds after the lock. Other companies may call a locked database a "frozen" database. Or, they may have a different way of using the term "freezing" the database, which compares more closely with other companies' terms of "close" or "soft lock." There are various processes that companies follow with respect to locking the database. The main rationale is that they must prove there was no bias introduced in the results before the blind is broken. Hence, they must document the point at which the database is considered to be of acceptable quality for the blind to be broken. Process is of vital importance when defining a metric. When looking at the time from last subject complete to database lock, this could be a different metric across companies if it is not carefully defined. In fact, the term "last subject complete" needs to be defined as well.

It is important to select relevant metrics that map to the goals of the corporation, department or site. The metrics must also have the correct units to allow for meaningful comparisons, even if these are across projects or process changes within a specific company.

Note

Example: An Inappropriate Metric

Many data management metrics are expressed as error rate per CRF page. But some case report form pages have just 10 data points while others have more than 100. Not only is this unit inappropriate for measuring productivity of data entry staff, it is also not a metric that translates well in terms of cross-trial comparisons nor to comparing the effectiveness of EDC/eCT systems for data collection to paper-based processes.

For metrics to be meaningful, they must be not only well-defined but also:

- Tied to measurable goals or objectives (e.g., corporate, departmental, project-specific)
- Relevant and useful
- Timely and accurate
- Reasonably available

- Monitored to and utilized for decisions (e.g., to determine modifications that are needed in a process)

Issues to Consider When Determining What Metrics to Track

Determining what to measure and defining appropriate metrics is not always straightforward. However, the time taken to do this is worthwhile. The steps include:

1. Deciding upon the goals.
2. Mapping the processes to see where and how these goals can be achieved.
3. Determining the measurements needed to show whether the goals are being met.
4. Defining the metric and the way the measurements are going to be taken, i.e., the factors or parameters that go into the calculations or assessments for the metric.

Most projects (or clinical trials) involve the management of five factors—scope, time, cost, risk, quality. Making a change to any one factor can easily have an impact on several other factors. In addition, the change will ripple through to the metrics that have been established for these factors. The most commonly defined metrics are typically for time, cost and quality. Scope can be thought of as the sum of all the products and services provided by a project. As such, metrics for scope typically need to be viewed in terms of the other factors, e.g., percent project completion versus time or cost. Risk metrics are also difficult to define in isolation. One option is to treat risk like scope and state metrics in terms of eliminating risk based on a specific expenditure of time or resources or both.

Defining metrics for time, cost and quality is more straightforward. They are also inter-related. For example, if a project team works to increase quality, this may increase the time or cost. If only time is measured, for example, this could give an idea of project quality and cost, but could also mask them. For this reason, identifying key metrics that include measurements of time, cost and quality will bring a more sound and valuable picture of the overall well-being or status of the project. For a given step or task in a project, however, it is not always necessary to track metrics for all five factors, but all five factors should be considered when planning a project.

Certain of the most valuable metrics may be difficult to obtain or compile. Sources for metrics may also be multiple and varied. The data for compiling them may exist in separate, disparate databases. The inherent difficulty in obtaining this information compromises not only timeliness but also compliance on the part of the project team, especially if they do not get feedback on the results in time for this to be useful. Reviewing outdated metrics decreases their meaning and their relevance to the current processes, and certainly the opportunities to act upon issues they raise. Metrics should be practical and collected in a timely manner.

One additional issue to point out is that different types of metrics are often not in sync. If the project/trial metrics report is taken at a different time than the financial report, it can lead to a guessing game about where the project stands and where it is headed.

> **Note**
>
> When managing studies across investigative sites, site personnel are frequently asked to send a fax or a post card or make a phone call to tell the sponsor or CRO how many patients were enrolled that week, how many have dropped out or discontinued and how many have completed. The data from these cards are then entered into another database used for tracking, after which enrollment graphs are developed. In a multi-center trial, it is potentially easy to over-enroll a trial or to have enrollment lagging for a couple of weeks before anyone can even detect the problem, much less rectify it. As always, the more times data are re-entered, the more opportunity there is to introduce error.

Metrics Drivers

Drivers are traits of the trial that will influence the metric and whether or not the goals will be achievable. They are components of the scope. When identifying a metric, also consider what the drivers are. For example, drivers for clinical trial costs could be the number of sites and subjects; these have a direct relationship to costs. A driver for enrollment cycle time will also be the number of subjects and sites; the more subjects involved, the longer the enrollment time period will be, unless more sites are added to compensate. The more complex the data (e.g., an in-patient oncology study vs. an out-patient balding study), the longer it will take to collect and monitor the data, hence, study complexity is a driver.

Key Metrics

As mentioned previously, metrics must be useful and relevant. Unless it is useful and relates to a project goal, why collect that metric? Metrics that are the most useful and meaningful can be called key metrics. It is also important not to collect so many metrics that the process becomes too cumbersome to encourage compliance or to accommodate timeliness of reporting. Therefore, a well-selected set of key metrics should provide an accurate indication of the process status or goal a manager or team is assessing. These key metrics are also called indicators. If a manager picks the right indicators, project status should be seen at a glance.

It is also interesting to keep in mind that these indicators may be different for different people. Depending on the role of the individual, certain measurements may or may not be meaningful. One way to deal with this is to provide different views of the information. Perhaps the CEO only wants the highest level of key metrics or indicators. Then, the data managers want the ones that indicate the status of what is occurring in their realm, the sites have metrics that are meaningful to them and the monitors have others that are most meaningful to them. The point is that everyone should track certain metrics, and an organization should have data to support many different ones, but those that are the most relevant or meaningful to one manager may be different from those most relevant to another. In an ideal situation, detailed metrics collected should support the highest level metrics. They should build on each other and not be separate sets of data. Those collecting the metrics should be aware of how their metrics are contributing to top-level goals.

Practical Metrics

Difficulty of collection also influences decisions on which metrics to collect, but the difficulty of collecting a certain metric should not prevent us from trying to collect it. The typical industry metrics—usually cycle times derived from dates when certain events occurred—are also relatively easy to collect. The clinical trials industry has very little accurate data on the more difficult-to-collect metrics such as actual costs or resource utilization. Accurate and useful cost/resource measurements are associated with activities or functions that require personnel time. CROs or companies that use CROs typically have the best information on costs in our industry. They track the time they spend on activities they complete for each of their sponsors.

But there is a tradeoff. If something is too difficult to collect, it may not be worth the added time spent. For example, time should be tracked in units that make sense such as hours, not minutes. Or, other metrics may be more easily collected and actually be decent indicators regarding whether the goals are being met. For example, some companies track whether the budget is being met or how many full-time equivalents (FTEs) are on the project, rather than time spent in hours by each individual.

Standardizing Metrics Within the Industry

Once metrics are selected, definitions become critical, as we have discussed. Otherwise, comparisons cannot be made accurately from one trial to the next within a company and certainly not across companies within the industry. Benchmarking companies have made some progress on standardizing metrics that they report. These metrics are defined in advance so that the reporting companies provide data that can be compared across the industry. As discussed earlier, the few metrics routinely compared across companies in our industry generally pertain to cycle times and to paper-based trials. The information typically is retrospective, and companies are not always willing to share their metrics with each other unless a benchmarking company is involved so that their responses can be blinded.

Fortunately, there is interest among different companies to share electronic clinical trials experiences. This requires establishing a set of key metrics that would be useful to those participating and then defining them carefully. Such sharing of information could potentially work better if technology vendors and CROs become involved, since they often have direct access to the metrics and can take some of the responsibility off the shoulders of sponsors.

It is important to establish a metrics program that does not point fingers but makes continuous improvement a team effort. Sometimes it is difficult to get people to share metrics internally because they are afraid of appearing to place blame on different departments or people. If possible, within an organization, it may help to have the key metrics set and defined, but let each project team recommend its own project-specific goals relevant to these metrics and a plan for achieving each goal.

Electronic clinical trials offer a tremendous advantage over paper-based trials for collecting certain metrics, since many of them are produced as a by-product of the process. (In paper-based trials, this opportunity only exists once the data are entered into an operational database, which is far into the trial and after the point when many project metrics are most needed. For this reason, most companies have a project management database that is separate from the operational database, thus requiring redundant data entry and reconciliation.) Sharing of eCT metrics can also help in standardizing these metrics and their definitions across the industry such that comparisons can be made for new technologies and processes.

Metrics for Assessing Electronic Clinical Trials

With a goal of comparing paper-based and eCT metrics, workshops have been held in the United States, Spain and France, with attendees representing pharmaceutical and biotech companies, CROs, IRBs, consulting firms, technology providers and others from the industry. A compilation of results from these workshops is included below as a sample set of goals and key metrics for the purpose of assessing the success of applying new technologies to clinical trials. It is also a starting point for the industry to create common metrics and definitions and begin to standardize these. It is critical to have baseline comparison metrics, so it is never too soon to begin a metrics collection effort.

Goals for Implementing eClinical Trial Strategies

- Shorten the drug development cycle
- Obtain cleaner data earlier (near real time)
- Improve access to information
- Enhance subject safety; facilitate safety monitoring
- Increase productivity; improve site performance; facilitate monitoring
- Decrease the cost of clinical trials
- Decrease paper; eliminate manual processes
- Simplify processes; eliminate the collection of superfluous data
- Streamline regulatory submissions

Comparative Key Metrics for eCT vs. Paper-Based Trials

As mentioned earlier, there is a real interplay among quality, time and cost when conducting a project. It is important when tracking metrics to understand their meaning and how they may have an impact on other metrics. Identifying key metrics that include measurements of quality, time and cost will provide a clearer picture of the overall well-being or status of the project. Examples of typical metrics for time, cost and quality that would pertain to comparisons of eCT vs. paper-based trials are listed below.

Time

- Protocol approval to first subject enrolled
- First subject enrolled to last subject enrolled
- Last subject complete to database lock
- Subject visit date to data accessible by sponsor
- Time to resolve a query; time to obtain clean data for a particular visit or subject

Cost

[Note: Cost is calculated by multiplying the time by the salary for that individual/functional group, including an appropriate overhead factor.]

- Overall trial cost (budgeted vs. actual)
- Resource requirements by type for specified activities (e.g., hours or FTE for monitors, data managers, technology providers, etc., for the planning period, training, study conduct, study closeout)
- Time spent to complete certain tasks (e.g., entry of data or monitoring of data for a specified visit)

Quality

- Number of queries on incoming data (with a denominator of data fields, not CRF pages)
- Number of edit checks firing or number of queries on specific data fields
- Number of protocol violations
- Number of protocol amendments

Other Useful Comparative Metrics

- Technology performance (e.g., time to enroll a subject or time between screens)
- Number of process steps eliminated without compromising quality
- "Inline" status information (e.g., graphs showing actual subject enrollment rate vs. planned rate; percentage of total data outstanding vs. the plan; data query rates and outstanding queries)

- Adverse events per site and/or per subject visit
- Time from protocol approval to a go/no-go decision (continue the trial, accelerate the next trial or stop a trial due to safety issues or lack of efficacy)
- Subjective assessments by investigator site personnel and project teams (e.g., eClinical Trials vs. EDC vs. paper processes)

Please also refer to the process maps in "Metrics for Assessing Newly Introduced Technology" in Chapter 4.

Advantages of eClinical Trials for Collecting Metrics

The collection of metrics in electronic clinical trials has several distinct advantages over the paper process:

1. Many metrics can be gathered automatically through an electronic technology system, including time and date of subject enrollment, data collection and query resolution. The time between certain actions can also be automatically calculated to produce cycle time measurements. Time and date stamps are recorded for these actions within the computer system, and a record of who logged into the system when the activities occurred is created.
2. Metrics can be available in real time or near real time, allowing for appropriate and timely interventions when they indicate that the trial is off-track.
3. Because much of the information from metrics is produced automatically via the computer system, this minimizes errors, inconsistencies and compliance issues.
4. Metrics can be tracked per data field or data item, rather than per case report form page, thus providing a more relevant and accurate denominator for cross-study or cross-company comparisons.

Letting the Metrics Work for the Team

Performance data that identify problem areas can lead to performance improvements in both currently active and future studies. By correcting performance problems quickly as a study progresses, costs and delays caused by preventable problems can be kept to a minimum. This is a project manager's nirvana. Those involved in assuring patient safety are also in desperate need of high quality data near real time.

Clinical trial metrics can show how well an investigative site is performing. For example, there should be minimal or no delays between a subject's visit and when visit data are collected electronically. The investigator with certain data or error rates outside of a normal distribution range is of concern. A higher incidence of adverse events during a certain visit across subjects may indicate a safety issue with a drug. Trend analyses can look at patterns to show which sites should be monitored more closely. Providing statistical performance data to CRAs or project managers as a trial progresses will help them identify problem areas and will also give them objective information to use if it is necessary to show an investigator or coordinator that a problem exists at a site.

Metrics can be used for management of functions, especially when they allow "drill-down" to the actual data. A CRA or a clinical project manager might identify a site or a CRA with a large number of outstanding queries. By drilling down into the data itself, it should be possible to actually identify individual outstanding queries and determine whether any pattern exists—for example, a problematic data item or CRF question. This type of information allows meaningful and timely interventions. With consistent and comparative data, a clinical trial team can proactively apply changes to the trial while it is in progress. The availability of better data faster permits in-depth questions such as:

- Are the data collection questions well-phrased or are some easily misinterpreted?
- Are site personnel and monitors adequately trained on the protocol and the system?
- What is the quality of the patient data?
- Are the automatic edit checks sufficiently and appropriately implemented, or are they over-implemented?
- Are the activities occurring per the scheduled clinical trial plan?

Reports on metrics data for study teams and management, presented visually, are critically important when trying to make effective use of the metrics data. Reports may show data trends, outliers, enrollment rates, distribution of adverse events across sites, cycle times or other useful information. Metrics should also indicate, for project management purposes, compliance with the project plan. For example, is the enrollment rate on target (i.e., actual versus planned at a given point in time)? Are the patient visits occurring on schedule? For such measurements and reports it is critical that there be goals, i.e., that there be targets or "planned" dates or measurements as well as actuals in the system. These reports or views can then be complemented with root cause analyses to identify underlying issues and a process that allows continuous improvement.

Conclusion

New technologies and electronic clinical trials make it possible to follow clinical trial status in a much more thorough and timely fashion than ever possible in the past. However, in order to maximize the value of metrics collection, it is critical that metrics be defined at the start of the project and that careful attention be given to what is actually measured. It is also important to have baseline metrics or planned/anticipated values for comparison. To make the most of metrics, identify those that are the indicators of established goals. What is a key metric may vary depending on the role of the individual using the metrics. Consequently, it is important that metrics be collected that support all the team members. It is important to pay attention to the process and to leverage new technologies to facilitate collection and viewing of these indicators. If metrics are available and assessed in near real-time (comparing them to a baseline and/or target goal), then time-critical decisions can be made sooner and modifications implemented in a more timely manner.

7

Performing Electronic Clinical Trials in Accord with Regulations

Objectives

- Define the intent of 21 CFR, Part 11 (the Rule) and list related regulatory guidance for electronic clinical trials (eCTs).
- List three types of signing accepted for electronic records and the standard for acceptance of electronic clinical trial (eCT) records by the FDA.
- Understand the central issues with respect to regulatory adherence in an electronic clinical trial so as to be able to plan and execute an electronic clinical trial (eCT) in accord with current regulation and guidance.

It is clear today that the regulatory agencies themselves are driving the industry toward eCTs. Clinical trials conducted by pharmaceutical companies and manufacturers of medical devices are subject to rules issued and enforced in the United States by the Department of Commerce and the Food and Drug Administration (FDA). In Europe, the European Union (EU) issues directives, which may be adopted in common, or nations may enact regulations independently. Certain member nations have independent laws and regulations that affect clinical research, approvals and marketing of medical devices and drugs.

While news and business publications seem to portray drug companies and regulators as adversaries, pharmaceutical companies and the FDA generally realize they are on the same side. Neither wants a bad drug marketed or a good drug delayed. The key to making both sides happy is to ensure data integrity so that the scientific decisions about efficacy and safety, and the medical decisions about when and how to use pharmaceuticals, are made from findings that can be trusted.

In the United States, the FDA recognized that the eCTs needed to have regulations and guidance in order for developers of the software and computer systems to design such systems with confidence. So, the FDA spent six years proposing and soliciting "comments" from industry and then deliberating. The result, generated while David Kessler was commissioner of the U.S. Food and Drug Administration [FDA] and Gerald Meyer was Acting Director of the Center for Drug Evaluation and Research [CDER], was what is now well known as "Part 11" or 21 CFR 11 (Code of Federal Regulations, Section 21, Part 11). (See Appendix E.) This regulation (The Rule), which became effective on August 20, 1997, sets out the rules for "electronic records" that may be submitted to the FDA, also known as "the Agency." The United States and the FDA have generally been the leaders in establishing these regulations; hence, this chapter focuses on FDA regulatory requirements for conducting eCTs. As of this writing, it appears that systems and processes compliant with FDA requirements will also meet privacy and research quality regulations issued by the EU and the International Committee on Harmonisation (ICH).

Other regulations or guidances that need to be considered in light of conducting eCTs are the Health Insurance Portability and Accountability Act of 1996, or HIPAA; European Union Directive on Privacy; FDA Guidance on Computerized Systems Used in Clinical Trials (CSUCT) (See Appendix F); and FDA Guidance for Electronic Submissions, which is not available in its updated version as of this writing.

Agency Aim in Creating 21 CFR 11

The Agency's aim with 21 CFR 11 was to encourage adoption of computerized systems in clinical research and realization of their benefits by setting the standards for systems handling electronic records. The FDA states that the final Rule was "…intended to permit the widest possible use of electronic technology."

The FDA's objectives in setting forth the Rule are stated in the FDA Guidance, CSUCT, and in the Rule (three pages) and a "preamble" stretching to 36 pages in the March 20, 1997, Federal Register. The Rule can be found at www.fda.gov under "Code of Federal Regulations, Section 21 Part 11."

Intent and Requirements of 21 CFR 11

The intent of creating this set of regulations was to "set forth the criteria under which the Agency considers electronic records, electronic signatures, and handwritten signatures executed to electronic records to be trustworthy, reliable, and generally equivalent to paper records and handwritten signatures executed on paper."

In other words, 21 CFR 11 entitled "Electronic Records; Electronic Signatures" establishes what a system for handling electronic records must do in order for the FDA to consider the system adequate for submitting electronic records in place of paper records. The Rule sets down in only three pages all the steps required by the FDA in order to assure that electronic records it receives are at least as good as the paper records it has been accepting.

Scope of The Rule

The Rule applies to all electronic records (… "records in electronic form that are created, modified, maintained, archived, retrieved or transmitted, under any records requirements set forth in Agency regulations"). The Rule does not apply to "paper records that are, or have been, transmitted by electronic means."

Electronic Signatures

Signatures have long been used to authenticate records. People recognize that they can be held accountable for agreements, actions, deeds, etc., which they have signed, and many records that the Agency requires must be signed or initialed. How does one sign an electronic record with a keyboard and a mouse? The FDA decided to accept three ways of signing:

1. **Digital signature:** This is a type of electronic signature that relies on a unique combination of at least two "identification components." Usually these are a login ID, which can be known by others, and a password, which should be completely private.
2. **Biometric signature:** This is a second type of electronic signature that is linked to an individual's identifying physical features or specific "repeatable actions." Examples would include retinal scans and systems that identify an individual by automatically matching handwriting during signing.
3. **Handwritten signature:** This is the traditional handwritten signature, and it is not an electronic signature. It cannot be executed with a keyboard and a mouse, but "devices" such as touch screens or pads that preserve the act of signing with a pen or stylus can do the trick.

The main achievement in signing electronic records either electronically or with the handwritten signature is to "link" the signature to the record itself. With paper CRFs, the physical properties of the paper keep the ink of the signature together with the data on the same piece of paper (or physically connected book of pages of paper). An electronic method of preserving the same linkage must be in place in order for signed electronic records to have acceptable integrity (to be as trustworthy as paper ones).

The Rule does not itself specify which actions or electronic records must be signed. The Rule establishes that electronic signatures can take the place of any signing or initialing requirements set forth in predicate rules (all other regulations in place that cover records to be submitted to the Agency) for electronic records. However, any such electronic records must themselves meet the requirements of the Rule and must therefore have been created, modified, maintained or transmitted only via systems that also meet the requirements of the Rule. Furthermore, even in cases where predicate rules do not require signing, the Agency clearly sets forth in the preamble to the Rule that it understands that electronic records might be signed whether or not such signing is required. Signing is a good way to attribute actions on electronic records by individuals, and it helps to authenticate them.

Regulatory Considerations in Planning an Electronic Clinical Trial

Know the regulations. This simple statement has many implications. The implementation of an electronic clinical trial must be compliant with regulations. Such compliance can only be accomplished by designing and planning the trial to meet the regulations. Below, we review how each step in planning and executing an electronic clinical trial must conform to FDA regulations.

Since the regulations were intended to preserve for electronic clinical trials the trustworthiness of an acceptable paper system, the prudent trial designer will start on the same page as the FDA starts. The regulation flowed from the objective of data quality and integrity as central principles. Thus, if you have the same notions of data integrity and quality as the FDA, then decisions about systems and processes for executing an eCT can flow with confidence from that understanding. The FDA makes this easy by publishing its understanding of data quality and integrity.

Data integrity: As stressed by Dr. Stan Woolen, head of the FDA office of Science and Research, in a presentation to the Drug Information Association [DIA] in 1999 on source documents, the keys to data integrity are in the mnemonic "ALCOA," which also appears in a different order in the Guidance for Computerized Systems Used in Clinical Trials (April, 1999) (CSUCT). The letters stand for:

- Attributable
- Legible
- Contemporaneous
- Original
- Accurate

The specific steps in adherence are given later in this chapter, but it is essential to focus on the intent of the regulations, not simply the details of specific provisions. ALCOA is the cornerstone of the regulations, but doesn't appear literally in its provisions. That's why the FDA orients readers of the

Guidance for Computer Systems Used in Clinical Trials [CSUCT, Office of Regulatory Affairs (ORA) April 1999] in the second paragraph of its introduction:

> *FDA established the Bioresearch Monitoring (BIMO) Program of inspections and audits to monitor the conduct and reporting of clinical trials to ensure that data from these trials meet the highest standards of quality and integrity and conform to FDA's regulations. FDA's acceptance of data from clinical trials for decision-making purposes is dependent upon its ability to verify the quality and integrity of such data during its onsite inspections and audits. To be acceptable the data should meet certain fundamental elements of quality whether collected or recorded electronically or on paper. Data should be attributable, original, accurate, contemporaneous, and legible. For example, attributable data can be traced to individuals responsible for observing and recording the data. In an automated system, attribution could be achieved by a computer system designed to identify individuals responsible for any input.*

System Validation

As quality engineers know, quality must be managed. One cannot have data integrity and quality in an eCT unless the underlying system for capturing the data, and for displaying, cleaning, reviewing, recovering and archiving the trial data has been validated. This is called system validation. The principle behind system validation is that the system does what it is intended to do. The Rule requires that persons who perform eCTs, "employ procedures and controls designed to ensure authenticity, integrity and, when appropriate, the confidentiality of electronic records…" The Agency thus establishes a high-level objective for what the system must be intended to do. It also sets forth another general requirement for electronic records that such procedures and controls should "…ensure that the signer cannot readily repudiate the signed record as not genuine." The Rule then specifies several such "procedures and controls" needed to satisfy the objectives of authenticity, integrity and "non-repudiation." The first of these is system validation. Persons who will act on electronic records in an eCT must do so with systems validated "… to ensure accuracy, reliability, consistent intended performance, and the ability to discern invalid or altered records." An auditor must be able to compare what the system does with what is documented as the intent for the system performance. Thus, in order for systems to be validated there must be documents that set forth in detail how they are intended to perform and a matching set of documents that demonstrate that the systems perform in the intended fashion. The validation of underlying computer systems used to process electronic records is discussed by FDA in its Draft Guidance for Industry (21 CFR Part 11; Electronic Records; electronic Signatures Validation, August 2001). At this point in performing an eCT the trial planner and designer will have audited the underlying system to be used and will have confirmed that it is validated. Thus the trial planner and designer may then turn to consider how to ensure the quality and data integrity for the particular trial.

There must be certain content in the Requirements Specification in order for an eCT to meet the regulations. For each eCT there must be a document that specifies how the clinical and operational managers of that eCT intend it to be implemented. If one is preparing to manage an eCT, it will be helpful to have a list of elements that should be in an eCT Requirements Specification so that the system used to act on electronic records in the trial can be validated and compliant with the Rule. In practice, the part of the Specification pertaining to compliance with the Rule may be written or obtained from a technology provider who supplies the system. Additional trial-specific requirements (all eCTs must comply with the Rule) may be combined with or supplemental to those pertaining to the Rule. Such a list of elements to be specified during planning can be found in Appendix D.

Planning and Design Steps for Meeting Regulations with an Electronic Clinical Trial

1. Develop a Requirements Specification.
The requirements specification is a crucial and indispensable planning document because it indicates what the intended operation of a particular trial is. For regulatory purposes, a requirements specification should be created before the system is customized for the trial and should meet the following recommendations:

Good system specification leads to good system design.

- The eClinical Requirements Specification document itself should be under version control.
- All system documentation related to the trial should be subject to change control procedures, and an audit trail must be maintained to document "time-sequenced" development or modification of the system, if any, during the trial.

Itemization of all system components.

- Audit or qualify any third-party software, server(s), client(s).
- Specify (and standardize if possible) the data to be included in electronic records (fields, tables) and the appearance and layout of such records.
- Clinical Data Interchange Standards Consortium [CDISC] standard. (See Chapter 10.)
- Corporate standards.

Edit check specifications.

- All edit checks intended to operate during the trial should be specified in the eCT Requirements Specification so that they can be validated.
- Point-of-entry edit checks should be designed carefully. They are very useful for error reduction and data quality. Generally such edit checks are best used to detect obviously wrong or impossible entries, but they should not prevent entry of unexpectedly large or small values, nor guide researchers to enter data that will confirm the hypothesis under test.
- Edit checks may "fire" locally on submission of a record, or they may be run at the server after the record is stored centrally.

Archiving electronic data and support for retrieval.

- Plan from the beginning how data, trial-related documentation and trial "reconstruction" will be accomplished. The Rule stipulates that electronic records must be retained (and be "readily" retrievable electronically) for as long as required for the equivalent paper record. For the FDA, the minimum retention period for records in support of a submission to the Agency is two years after a trial concludes. In Europe, retention requirements may stretch to fifteen years. Archiving electronic records for electronic recovery and trial reconstruction is not easy because of the ongoing evolution of hardware, software and storage technology. For example, data stored on 5.25-inch floppies is becoming unreadable in the 21st century because such drives are simply disappearing.
- The archived electronic records themselves must be secure and protected so that they remain accurate.

Plan for electronic source instead of paper source.

- Guidance (CSUCT) stipulates that source documents "should be retained to enable a reconstruction and evaluation of the trial."
- Guidance (CSUCT) also stipulates that "when original observations are entered directly into a computerized system, the electronic record is the source document." Electronic diary data is often electronic source.
- Sites need to have a source document verification (SDV) SOP.
- Sites need to confirm that the SDV process will work with the planned trial.

Security and audit trail design.

- The Rule requires that all users of the implemented system who may act upon electronic records must be identified and trained. Such identification and training must be documented.
- The audit trail must be secure and computer-generated.
- The audit trail must record each action (entry, edit or modify, or "deletion") on an electronic record. Each record in the audit trail must include the time stamp of the action, and attribute the action to a specific individual.

Access controls.

- Ensure that specifications exist for how access to the system will be limited and how distribution of and access to the system documentation will be controlled.
- If digital signatures will be used to control access to the system, specify that users will "sign" at beginning of sessions if using digital signatures.
- Other access controls, such as codes to be entered in order to bring up screens for data entry, may be useful if you will be using handwritten signatures to authenticate data.

Authenticity controls.

- ID and password management must be specified for all planned users of the system who will act on electronic records under their electronic signatures. A system must be in place during execution of the trial to document that each user has been identified and that they have agreed that their electronic signature is the "legally binding equivalent" of their handwritten signature.
- A policy and process must be in place to hold users of the system accountable for actions performed under electronic signatures.
- If electronic signatures will be used, a certificate for all planned users in the trial should also be on file with the FDA that establishes that an organization including such users intends that electronic signatures will have the full legal weight of handwritten signatures.

Privacy Protection.

- Plan for privacy protection and test that access and authority controls fulfill the privacy requirements. Establish which study personnel shall be entitled to know the patient names and contact information and stipulate that all others will not see patient names or other personal information. Such matters need to be spelled out in the informed consent so that research data can retain regulatory integrity, yet be able to be electronically analyzed, transferred, published, etc. Generally this should be accomplished by reliance on the consent form as a waiver of the myriad of privacy protection issues that might be in place.

- Companies can undertake certification as a "safe harbor" for private information. This is a self-certification based on auditable requirements. The safe harbor act provides some stiff penalties for violations. Safe harbor certification does not serve in place of waivers and authorizations to disclose private health information, which should still be part of informed consent forms signed by eCT subjects.

2. Create a Traceability Matrix.

The technology provider(s) of any system to be used in an eCT should provide a traceability matrix to the trial sponsor and/or be audited by the sponsor to ensure that they have system documentation that details how each specific regulatory requirement is met by the system(s) that will be used in the trial to act on electronic records. A traceability matrix showing the component of the Rule (regulatory requirement) next to the documentation of how the system/vendor is compliant with this component is a useful means to ensure this. Reviewing such a matrix during the planning stages of a trial will help ensure data integrity and extend the value of the trial data. Please refer to Appendix D for a sample traceability matrix.

3. Develop a Validation Plan.

The validation plan is for documenting the testing that must occur to ensure that the system performs the way it is intended to perform. All of this testing and conformance to the regulations must be documented within the validation documentation. The following considerations are important:

- Testing (as detailed in the validation plan) must be completed prior to enrolling the first clinical trial participant.
- The aim is quality of the data (trustworthy records), so documenting must be done: General auditing principles are:
  a. Intent (requirements)
  b. Employee actions (training and agreements done and documented)
  c. Results (Show that the eClinical System and process fulfill the intent; this requires records of intent and results of testing.)
- The cornerstone of validation is proof that the system works as intended. Trial-specific and comprehensive "intents" must be documented, and test results must show that operations match "intended."
  – Complete specifications.
  – Test records (Each requirement is met either by being tested as confirmed by an executed test document or by documented process.)
  – Evaluation (Documentation of the review and decision to deploy the system and move into the trial execution phase.)
- Plan for mid-course corrections. Validate that the eCT system can support the development, testing, validation, and deployment of changes in the protocol. As per regulations, any changes to either the trial-specific

system or its documentation, to the system documentation, or to the process of conducting the trial must be under change control. Such changes also must be recorded with an audit trail, and with documentation sufficient to reconstruct them. A useful capability is for a "production test" version of each deployed study to be maintained for the purpose of analyzing any problems in the currently deployed study and for developing, testing, and validating any changes.

> **Note**
> Undocumented perfection is like magic; it can be admired, but it can't be trusted.

4. Develop an Archiving Plan that Supports Data Retrieval.

In order to reconstruct the trial in the future during an audit, some planning is necessary. To that end, a plan should be written that specifies what documentation (all trial-specific testing, system and supporting documentation, the eCT Requirements Specification, trial data and metadata, protocol requirements, etc.) will be archived. The plan should also document how the archived documents and data will be used to reconstruct the trial for ready and electronic retrieval of the electronic records.

Regulatory Considerations While Executing an Electronic Clinical Trial

Clinical trial managers will generally have participated in the planning, and the above-mentioned requirements documents will make execution relatively easier than with a clinical trial for which data are collected and processed by traditional paper methods. This is because paper has well-known limitations, one of which is flexibility of completing forms (who and when). Planning for the more constrained case of eCT execution tends to force thinking, training and communication to occur that simply doesn't happen when trials are executed using paper for data collection and management. At the point where the switch is to be thrown to bring an eCT system into operation to conduct a trial, which we refer to as "deployment," the following elements should be in place in order to ensure that the trial can be reconstructed from its documents and that it will be conducted in compliance with regulations.

Data Integrity

eCTs result in datastreams of electronic records. While regulations do not require daily inspection of such datastreams, doing so will show a commitment to data integrity and trustworthiness of electronic records. Make daily checks a part of your plan. The following attributes of data integrity are worth inspecting based on the FDA Guidance on Computerized Systems Used in Clinical Trials ("To be acceptable the data should meet certain fundamental elements of quality whether collected or recorded electronically or on paper. Data should be attributable, original, accurate, contemporaneous, and legible.") In addition, the Rule requires procedures and controls "designed to ensure the authenticity, integrity, and, as appropriate, the confidentiality of electronic records from the point of their creation to the point of their receipt." This would obviously include the entire period of execution of an eCT as well as during the retention period. Generally a trial manager would rely on the audit of the system performed before the trial starts in order to confirm that during trial execution the system will impose appropriate encryption, access controls, authority checks and other features sufficient to make a compelling story about data integrity.

Attributable

- Actions on records should be made by trained individuals. Check for presence of such training documentation. Each company needs to specify in an SOP where the training documentation is stored; an auditor will check the archive.
- Signature agreements should be in place for all signers. Keep signature agreements and identity certifications and include them in the archive. Ensure that the signing affidavits are appropriate for actions being taken at the appropriate times and places.
- Assess the actions being taken on electronic records to see that a logical and consistent chain of evidence supports the responsibility and accountability for those actions (non-repudiation).

Legible

For eCTs, this is easy. Datastream monitoring might detect logical inconsistencies in legible data, however, and resolving such inconsistencies as soon as they occur can increase data integrity.

Contemporaneous

Data entry into electronic records in eCTs still is mostly accomplished by manual transcription from paper source documents at the site. Since such data entry can be tracked centrally as soon as it is done, the management of this process can be quite timely. In order to maximize this aspect of guidance on data integrity, managers of eCTs should use the systems to track and encourage submission of contemporaneous data by sites. The bull's eye on the target for contemporaneous trial data can be hit when data are captured as electronic source and submitted at the time the measurement or assessment is done. Contemporaneous review of data is enabled by contemporaneous entry. Early review enables data problems to be raised (queries) and resolved before memories and context have faded. In addition, comments and annotations made by individuals on electronic records during the trial can be checked to see whether issues are emerging as the trial proceeds that were unexpected and for which planning was inadequate. Contemporaneous review enables close management of a trial, and thus supports the manager's objective of maintaining data integrity as well as compliance with the protocol.

Original

Technology providers can help avoid entry of duplicate data by edit checks that ensure each patient is unique and that data entry occurs in the expected sequence. Datastream monitoring can add significantly to data integrity by tracking and ensuring that sites follow the plan for data entry that defines which forms and fields will be entered as eSource or by transcription from paper source documents. Monitoring visits can focus on ensuring that sites possess and retain original source documents.

Accurate

Managers derive the expected benefit here from their technology providers if the specification, testing and validation of edit checks have been properly planned and documented prior to deployment. The system used to enter, access, review, query, edit and correct the electronic records can:

- Minimize incorrectly entered data (use edit checks)
- Prevent mistakes from being improperly corrected or changed (record all changes in an audit trail)
- Help detect problems and inconsistencies early (perform datastream monitoring)

Trial Reconstruction

The auditing practices and guidance documents establish an important constraint on trial execution. eCTs must be done with systems and procedures that ensure creation of all the records needed to "Reconstruct" the trial. These include:

- Who did what when? (Record all actions on electronic records via a computer-generated audit trail, record all changes to the system or documentation via an audit trail.)
- At any given time, who executed the trial, and what training and authorization did they have? This common sense issue can be supported by a tracking "table of authorities" that documents roles and "privileges" (editing, entry, etc.) for all study staff using the system to act on electronic records.
- What did the patients have to do? (This is set by documents and practices, including the protocol, study plans, electronic diaries, all forms completed directly by patients, together with any constraints and tasks.)

- How were the data collected? (Trial reconstruction must reveal which data had been transcribed from paper, which data had been entered as eSource, the roles of individuals who acted on it, the actions of users of the system when they collected or edited data and the views of the users.)
- What changes were made as the trial progressed?
- Reconstruction must show the edits and the audit trail and any change management documentation for midstream changes to the system, protocol and procedures bearing on the final data.
- How were security and privacy ensured?
  - Interim data delivery. (Controls on access to data, controls and content of graphs and tables used to manage the trial.)
  - Treatment/privacy of identifying data specified in HIPAA or in the EU privacy directive for international trials:
  - All signed electronic records and data summaries.
  - Signed electronic records from confidential signers (patients, family). Managers should plan, test and document that such records and summaries display blinded electronic records without a "signature manifestation," which would otherwise be required to "include the printed name of the signer."
  - Final data delivery. (To whom, how and when data were delivered to the sponsor, report writers and analysts.)

Archiving and Retention of Data and Records

The archive should specify the intended path for reconstructing the trial from the data contained in it. Possibilities include:

- The "Dynamic" solution whereby the reconstruction of the trial proceeds by running the EDC system used originally to capture the data and process it. This solution may sound appealing, but becomes very difficult to achieve without mothballing hardware, software and systems. Network architecture evolution will probably prevent reconstruction of a fully distributed trial years after it is completed.
- Workable archiving solutions that permit computerized facilitation of examination and analysis of records in the full context of the trial can be accomplished by using ASCII character-based solutions, e.g., PDF files to show the appearance of eCRFs and planning documents, XML datastores (such as the CDISC Operational Data Model) to preserve data, metadata, and signed actions.

As in the regulations set forth above, the Rule requires preserving data integrity from the point and time of capture throughout the retention period. This can be accomplished using XML technology in conjunction with certified copies and signature linkage. Other solutions are possible. Managers have the obligation of assessing the archival solution in terms of its compliance with regulations.

Regulatory Demands on the Sites

General Considerations

Sponsors are fundamentally responsible for the conduct of the electronic clinical trial, and they generally audit the technology provider(s) in support of this responsibility. Sponsors set forth the basic requirements for data to be captured and the roles and obligations that trial personnel shall have. At present, the experience of technology providers, with eCTs, is often greater than that of sponsors. This fact leads sponsors to rely on such providers to sharpen the requirements and to help with the planning of trials. The technology providers perform the validation testing and documentation for eCTs except under conditions where the sponsor is using its own technology, not a third party, so the sponsor has to meet these requirements and actually executes the trial without outsourcing the EDC.

Sponsors must understand that to the extent they engage a technology provider in a trial to capture, access, edit, correct and maintain electronic records, the preparation and maintenance of such records (i.e., the content of data fields and the obligation for accuracy) remain with the site. Generally this is specified in the study requirements documents pertaining to the trial and is ensured by implementation and validation of the system used to execute the trial.

Data Retention

Sponsors retain the complete clinical trial archive materials, including all documentation needed to reconstruct a trial. This includes electronic casebooks, the datasets, validation documentation and reconstruction guidance as well as certified copies of the archived materials sent to each site. Sponsors are responsible for setting the retention periods in accordance with regulatory requirements for such trial archives and for ensuring that the technology provider can preserve the electronic records during the entire retention period. The records also must be available for trial reconstruction as needed during this period.

Privacy Protection

The data set used by the sponsor for analysis can fulfill privacy protection if it does not contain any personal information. The system used for trial conduct cannot meet the demands for data integrity and being attributable without documented assurance that the patients truly existed and were duly enrolled. Thus, the system used to execute the trial must have other controls to protect privacy. Analysis of completely anonymous data, however, may reasonably be done after validated transfer. Note that the Health Insurance Portability and Accountability Act [HIPAA] and EU Privacy directives envision a sunset clause in waivers of disclosure of personal health information. Subjects may be entitled to know when the access of auditors and study personnel to private information will come to an end. It would therefore be prudent to establish a sunset requirement in the interest of maximizing privacy. Such a requirement would also permit design and validation of a system to ensure the requirement is met.

Certification for use of Electronic Signatures

Sponsors may elect to submit a certification concerning use of electronic signatures under 21 CFR 11.100. The Agency offers the following example (item 119, preamble to the Rule). "Pursuant to Section 11.100 of Title 21 of the Code of Federal Regulations, this is to certify that [sponsor name] intends that all electronic signatures executed by our employees, agents, or representatives, located anywhere in the world, are the legally binding equivalent of traditional handwritten signatures." Note that such a certification would not apply to patients if such patients were to use electronic signatures to enter data in the form of self reports. Such patients are not employees, agents, or representatives of sponsors. Thus, in order to comply with 21 CFR 11.100 for patient signatures, a certification for use of digital signatures should be provided to the Agency for each patient.

Regulatory Demands on Technology Providers

General Considerations

Providers of technology for systems to conduct eCTs are paid by the sponsors. Usually sponsors establish eCT requirements stating that data are to be retained (accessible and maintained) by the site. In this sense, the technology provider may be hired by the sponsor specifically to be neutral concerning data content, and to ensure as a trusted third party that data cannot be changed by the Sponsor or by any other party that is not neutral. Sponsors and GCPs will require that the technology provider not execute any changes to data (except to the extent that such changes are executed under the instruction and consent of the site). During execution of trials in which hosting, back-up, telecommunications and network infrastructure are outsourced, the technology provider will act like a bank: it holds the data (money) on behalf of its client sites (account holders) who can alter the data (deposit, withdraw, correct) and who count on the technology provider (bank) to maintain the data (accounts) without fraudulent or untracked changes.

Access Controls

The access and authorization controls on the electronic records must be implemented by the technology provider and be approved under audit by the sponsor. The technology provider has the technical responsibility for compliance with the Rule and with other regulations concerning the integrity of electronic records and the systems that act on them.

Stability of System

Adequate processes and management consistency must be manifested by the technology provider to assure regulators that the system preserves integrity of data and electronic records. Sponsors can either ask for a validation report and/or conduct an audit on their own to make sure the system meets their own requirements.

Archiving and Retention of Data

As with the preceding responsibilities, the responsibility for data archiving also belongs with the technology provider. At present, computer sales persons appear on television regularly suggesting that scanning family photographs onto CDs will immortalize them. This is not true because systems for retaining data are still in rapid evolution, and recovery of data from older methods becomes progressively more difficult with time. Technology providers must ensure against such rotting of electronic data, and must proof archives throughout the retention period. Regulations do not stipulate that the technology provider must retain the archival materials on behalf of the sponsor, but certainly some clear provision for such retention must be made for each eCT.

Conclusion

If one sifts through the regulatory requirements worldwide and examines the systems for executing eCTs today, as we have in this chapter, the evidence supports a belief in the possibility of compliance. The requirements are multiple and varied, but they can be met. The prudent manager of eCTs must keep the equivalent of a substantial checklist in mind to ensure that each regulatory element is fulfilled. As expertise continues to build at the levels of the trial managers, the sponsor auditors, the FDA office of compliance and the technology vendors themselves, compliance will become an ordinary expectation.

From the scope, preamble and various DIA presentations it is clear that the Agency wants electronic data collection and submission. The scientific and regulatory reviewers and the archivists want reliable retention and retrieval. Scientists need to explore the data and form their conclusions more easily and with greater confidence. Examining the warning letters and 483 citations issued by the FDA that have appeared to date, one does not see any indication that the Agency is citing instances where fine interpretation of the regulations has been at issue. Instead, the Agency has cited such gross problems as: security lack, absence of system validation, no systematic change control documentation or process, no computer-generated audit trail capability, no process for holding users accountable for actions under digital signatures.

Agencies must accept records electronically by 2003 (Government Paperwork Elimination Act 1998). The FDA has said it will accept electronic records and signatures compliant with its standards as of August 1997. The real question is, "When will they not accept paper?" For years FDA personnel have complained of drowning in paper. It now appears that the office of submissions is writing a regulation to require electronic submissions in the future. Such submissions will be easier if the trials themselves are done as electronic clinical trials.

CHAPTER 8

Data Quality and Data Integrity

Objectives

- Define data integrity.
- Understand the challenges in defining and measuring data quality and be able to list five possible sources of error during data transformation.
- Identify three practical approaches that can be used to ensure capture of data that are accurate, consistent and reflect a patient's experience in a clinical study.
- Understand the relationships between data validation procedures and data quality.
- Recognize the need to balance the costs and risks with the likely outcomes in making data quality management decisions.

Standards-compliant eClinical trial technology can go a long way toward improving the conduct of clinical trials. It can streamline the capture and processing of clinical trial data, improve communications and lead to a dramatic reduction in the number of errors introduced into trial databases because of manual re-keying of data. Ultimately, however, understanding the issues relating to data quality, and taking them into account when planning and conducting the study, are most important in ensuring that the database used for regulatory submission accurately reflects the contents of source data. This chapter will review several key points to consider in planning for data quality and data integrity.

Definitions of Data Quality and Data Integrity

Although there is wide recognition of the importance of data quality, no industry standards or widely accepted definitions of quality data exist. Given the absence of these standards, data quality is usually defined based upon "fitness for use"—its ability to meet needs or expectations rather than conformity to a set of specifications. In the context of a clinical study, "fitness for use" means the data are able to meet the intent and needs of an investigator or reviewer. In other words, the study database must be able to support meaningful conclusions and interpretations. In practical terms, this means the database must document the relationship between the original study protocol and the procedures actually followed for the study, and must be able to support generation of analyses that will be useful to evaluate the study hypotheses. Because assessments of database quality are linked to the needs of the study and expectations of the user, the quality criteria may vary from one project to another.

The definition of data integrity is less ambiguous. It means that the content of the submission database matches that found in source data. 21 CFR Part 11 and the FDA guidance document on Computer Systems Used in Clinical Trials provide direction regarding management of data to ensure data integrity, but do not specify minimum acceptable criteria for data quality and completeness.

Error Sources

Data related to the patient experience in an investigative study undergo a series of transformations from the patient to presentation of study results. That transformation takes these steps:

- An observation or measurement is made.
- Measurement is recorded.
- Recording may be transcribed to a paper report form or worksheet.
- Data from form or worksheet are entered into an electronic system.
- Data are stored and managed in the electronic system.
- Data may be transferred from one electronic system to another (multiple times).
- Data are then transformed into raw analysis data sets.
- Raw data sets are converted into analysis-ready data structures.
- Analysis-ready data are used to generate the results output.

The danger is that errors or changes to the data can potentially be introduced at any point along the way. If many or substantive errors/changes are introduced, then the data may not accurately reflect the true patient experience with the product and may become less suitable for making an evaluation of a product's safety and efficacy.

The U.S. government has enacted a number of requirements, including 21 CFR Part 11 and guidance documents intended to ensure that systems and procedures are in place to protect against the introduction of errors or unintended changes to the data and to provide mechanisms to detect unintended changes. These regulations are fundamental to providing a high level of data integrity. Data-handling guidelines and other approaches are used in conjunction with the FDA regulations to ensure that the clinical data are of appropriate quality.

Basic Principles

A number of practical approaches are used to ensure capture of data that is accurate, consistent and reflects a patient's experience in a clinical study. They include:

- Creating a concise, straightforward protocol and clear data forms.
- Reviewing incoming data to insure consistency and integrity using standardized quality checks.
- Examining the database for variations in data completeness (frequency of missing values) and distribution of variable values across enrolling sites. Large variations from site to site may indicate inconsistency in thoroughness of data collection and in application of definitions.

One of the advantages of electronic data capture systems is that data validity and completeness checks can be incorporated into the point-of-care data collection systems. Real-time data validation of out-of-range values and missing key variable fields increase the likelihood that the data will be captured correctly. More complicated data checks that consider consistency across multiple forms and data sources—or across sites—may be performed after the data have been transmitted to the data center.

It is important to recognize that a data quality management plan focused entirely on ensuring the accuracy and reliability of individual data points may not provide an efficient or high value product. A massive comprehensive data validation effort, with each individual value for each patient checked for completeness, real-world values and logical inconsistencies, is extraordinarily costly and, if it delays database lock and decision making in development, it may also result in delays in getting the right treatments to the right patients. The number of data checks that can be performed is almost unlimited. In the absence of a rational strategy for database quality management, a great deal of resources and time may be needlessly expended in attaining a small incremental gain in data completeness. The way to avoid such unnecessary expenditures is to create a data quality plan.

Data Quality Plan

A data quality plan should reflect a thoughtful assessment of the study, an understanding of the likely impact of missing and/or discrepant data on the study results, and the methods available. These objectives define quality criteria that describe the accuracy and reliability or "fitness for use" of a database in terms of the overall goals of the clinical study.

Critical elements of the trial must be of the highest level of quality but may vary with the type and nature of the study. Critical elements typically include:

- Documentation of randomization for comparison to the allocation scheme.
- Data that describe whether patients meet inclusion and exclusion criteria.
- Primary endpoint measurements.

Additional criteria may be extremely important in particular types of trials. For example, in a trial with a non-inferiority hypothesis, a lack of adherence may invalidate the findings as opposed to merely reducing power (as is the case in a superiority trial). It is therefore essential, in the case of a non-inferiority trial, to ensure maximal adherence to the treatment assignments. And it's important to carefully assess when patients are on and off study medications and the reasons for adherence issues.

A common approach in the clinical research industry is defining a quality standard by arbitrarily setting an acceptable error rate and then monitoring the data to ensure that it meets this standard. For example, the target might be set at 50 errors per 10,000 fields overall. An in-house audit is then performed on a selected random sample of enrolled patients to document the frequency of errors and determine whether or not the database achieves the target error rate. Database listings are cross-checked against the case report form and corresponding data clarification forms or, ideally, the source documents. The discrepant or missing items are determined and divided by the number of responded fields to generate an error rate.

Some organizations set different standards for critical and non-critical variables—commonly ranging from zero to ten errors per 10,000 fields for critical variables and twenty to one hundred errors per 10,000 fields for non-critical variables. An extreme expectation is that the error rate for critical variables or in critical panels should be zero and that this can be achieved through 100% manual review. However, an error-free database is neither practical nor necessary for data to support meaningful conclusions and interpretations. The comprehensive data cleaning process required to ensure an error-free database is extremely costly—delaying an understanding of the safety and efficacy of investigational therapies. Because there is a great deal of limited guidance on how to define quality data, a great many resources and a great deal of time are often invested, many at considerable cost, in striving for an error-free database.

Data Inspection and Clarification

The following are representative of data commonly subjected to inspection and clarification. Data that are:

1. Essential for identification or categorization of patients.
2. Required for pre-specified primary or secondary efficacy analyses.
3. Described or detailed study drug administration.
4. Related to an adverse event report.
5. Provide key safety information related to compound.
6. Documented investigator's perception of relationship of adverse or clinical event to study drug.
7. Trigger cases for endpoint event review and or adjudication.
8. Used in definition of clinical endpoint events.

For data that do not meet any of the above criteria, data quality efforts may be focused on optimizing completeness and accuracy of data when case report forms are submitted, rather than clarification of missing or inconsistent data. On the other hand, some critical data components may actually have redundant checks. For example, inclusion and exclusion criteria may be checked at the time of randomization and through key elements of the case report form.

Evaluating the Database

Decision making on what to do if data are missing or inconsistent should be based on an evaluation of the ability of the study database to support conclusions and interpretation compared to that of an error-free (or completely clean) database.[1]*

When only a small fraction of records require change, corrections may have little impact on the aggregate or summary data. The small number of studies that are available suggest that the error rate can be quite high in studies with moderate to large sample sizes before a loss of power is observed.[2] In large studies it is unlikely that the presence of data inconsistencies that are randomly distributed across treatment arms will have an impact on the ability of the database to support reliable conclusions and interpretations. However, data cleaning may have an important impact on efficacy endpoints where missing values or errors may not be randomly distributed. This is because patients who have experienced morbid or fatal events may be more difficult to locate and assess.

---

* Please see Appendix A for endnotes

Conclusion

eClinical trial systems must include data quality management processes and systems to enable operational improvements in clinical trials. To recognize the best return on investment in clinical research dollars and effort, data quality efforts may be targeted to areas most prone to errors and those integral to the requirements of the project. This requires application of knowledge of where errors are likely to occur and where additional data or data corrections are likely and important. In many cases, metrics exist to help researchers predict the probability that data will change if it is queried. A process should be in place for balancing the costs and risks against likely outcomes in these decisions.

The Impact of eClinical Trial Technology on Safety Surveillance and IRBs

Objectives

- Describe the responsibilities of the parties involved in clinical trials.
- Discuss the problems of patient safety monitoring.
- Discuss how eClinical Trial technology can improve safety surveillance.
- Discuss the issues of patient privacy.

The ethical mandate imposed by the testing of unproven therapeutic agents on patients and volunteers makes safety the overwhelming objective in clinical trials. In the United States, the clinical trial process is highly regulated by the Food and Drug Administration [FDA] and the federal government for the protection of the public good. The process involves overview by the physician administering the drug, the medical monitor at the pharmaceutical company, the FDA, an Institutional Review Board [IRB] and, increasingly, by a Data Safety Monitoring Board [DSMB]. The interaction among these parties acts as a set of checks and balances to help assure the safety of clinical trial subjects and patients. As with many processes in the pharmaceutical industry, communications, notifications and data review are typically carried out by these organizations through cumbersome, paper-intensive mechanisms. These paper-based processes sometimes lead to crucial and dangerous delays in safety reviews. The introduction of electronic processes, data capture to electronic adverse event reporting and IRB procedures can reduce delays in communication of safety issues among investigators, monitors, sponsors and FDA.

Time Delay

A key to patient safety in clinical trials is access to current data. Typically, paper-based clinical trials introduce significant delays between the collection of data at a clinical site, and the availability of the data for review by medical monitors, IRBs, DSMBs and anyone else who has responsibility for ensuring patient safety in a clinical trial. This is illustrated in Figure 9-A. The straight line represents an idealized view of the collection of data at a site during the study. Once a study begins, patients are enrolled and data are collected in a linear fashion until the last patient is seen in the clinic for the last visit.

Various activities in completion, monitoring, data entry and data programming introduce significant delays in access to these data. The S-curve represents the subset of these data that is available for safety review at any moment. At any point during a trial, there is a significant differential between the collected data and the available data. Identification of important safety trends, such as seasonal or batch-related toxicities, could easily be missed for months because of the delayed data access. In contrast, data collected using Internet-based clinical data management systems can be immediately available for data review. Notification of safety monitors via email or beeper can be automated, and medical monitor, IRB and DSMB access to real-time data can be provided.

Responsibilities for Monitoring Patient Safety

A clinical trial conducted in the U.S. involves overview by the physician administering the drug, the medical monitor at the pharmaceutical company, government regulatory agencies and by an institutional or independent review board (IRB) or ethics committee with authority to oversee human research at a particular institution. The following sections will discuss some of the specific roles and responsibilities of the various personnel and organizations involved in a clinical trial, and the impact of electronic processes on their ability to monitor safety issues. Other countries have similar processes executed through committees and regulatory agencies analogous to those of the U.S.

The IRB

Patient safety considerations begin with the IRB. The IRB operates through the oversight of the U.S. Food and Drug Administration (FDA) and/or the Office for Human Research Protection (OHRP). An IRB consists of a minimum of five people, including at least one scientist, one nonscientist and one person not affiliated with the institution. Typically, IRBs include a community representative, ethics expert or religious leader. At academic institutions, an IRB is often located on-site, but non-academic investigative sites typically use central IRBs that may be located hundreds or even thousands of miles away.

An IRB is responsible for overseeing the administration of a clinical protocol at a particular site to ensure that patients are not exposed to undue risks, have been appropriately recruited and have been adequately informed of the risks and benefits by signing the informed consent document. On a drug not yet approved, no human subject research can be started, and no ongoing research can continue, without an IRB approval. The IRB has the responsibility for reviewing the protocol and study forms, approving the informed consent and conducting ongoing annual reviews of the research. In addition, the IRB has the responsibility for reviewing serious adverse events that have been reported to regulatory agencies, on an ongoing basis.

There is no expectation that IRBs will closely monitor safety in a clinical trial—that responsibility falls to the investigator and medical monitor. However, the review of information by the IRB must be efficient and carefully tracked to ensure that safety notifications are properly reviewed and that investigations continue without problems. In most settings, the IRB operates through a paper process—documents are collected and reviewed in paper form, and approvals are submitted back to investigators on paper.

To improve their quality and efficiency, IRBs can adopt fully electronic processes for their work. Starting with protocol submissions and informed consent approval, IRB workflow can be automated through the use of appropriate software. Approvals can be electronic, and subsequent annual reviews and adverse event notifications can occur electronically. A central database can provide access to any pertinent data about adverse events and protocol details. Computer software can efficiently manage all necessary information, including acknowledging and responding to sponsors, CROs and investigators. The result is a fully electronic IRB review, with the benefits of automated tracking and project management.

In fact, there is no reason why an IRB cannot utilize technology so that they can become virtual. Members of a virtual IRB would not have to be located in the same city or state. They could assemble for a meeting no matter where they were. Videoconferencing could link the members visually, allowing for full discussion of important matters before decisions are made.

Note

In one Internet-based clinical trials system used for a global clinical trial with over 20,000 subjects, the IRB had access to appropriate site records. In cases where there were any significant concerns, the IRB had the authority to put a hold on sites such that they could not enter data until the issue was resolved.

The Investigator

An investigator shares with IRBs and sponsors the responsibility for ensuring that study subjects are adequately protected. They are required to assure that the IRB reviewing the study is in compliance with federal regulations. Investigators must be appropriately qualified to conduct the research and are responsible for ensuring that the research is conducted according to the protocol as approved by the IRB.

The first interaction between the patient and the investigative physician that involves safety is the consent process for patients or subjects. The informed consent process must include ongoing, dynamic communication as new safety information becomes available or is desired. Newly identified adverse experiences may require updating of informed consent with IRB approval, and patients must be presented with the most recent version of the consent. There are typically several parties other than the principal investigator involved, such as nursing, scientific or medical staff. Keeping track of and maintaining paper-based communication among everyone so that consent information is up-to-date can be a slow, error-prone process. The consent process can be managed through clinical trial management software, enabling the investigator to efficiently file and log all IRB communications.

During the conduct of the trial, the investigator must identify, record and assess adverse events. The adverse event profile of a drug is a very important aspect of clinical research. Typically, these are recorded on paper CRFs, where any aggregation or cross-tabulation of adverse events would require significant work on the part of the investigator so that associations between patients and adverse events would only occur through serendipity or an astute investigator. The compilation of adverse events in an electronic data capture system can create a more efficient process for review of these events across all patients at a site. If an investigator has enrolled hundreds of patients during a year or more, that investigator could only truly assess trends in adverse events by electronic compilation.

Some or all serious adverse events (SAEs), depending on the study and location, must be reported to the sponsor and/or the IRB. Regardless of the specific requirements for reporting, the information required for evaluation of an adverse experience far exceeds the information typically included on a case report form. De-identified source data and extensive questions and commentary may be requested of the investigator to thoroughly characterize the event. Several software packages are available for the capture of this information at investigative sites and for the reconciliation of the data with the clinical trials (CRF-based) database. Special software can even be used to report this information directly to regulatory authorities and back to all IRBs involved in the trial. The application of computerized collection and distribution of the data can help the sponsor meet regulatory timelines in the reporting of such data and can make the eventual annual reports, summary reports and regulatory submissions a more automated process. IRBs can also be provided with a read-only login to the clinical trial data of patients. This allows direct reviews, when necessary, of safety data from a clinical trial. An IRB might want to use such a mechanism to help evaluate a reported adverse event. The availability of such information can eliminate weeks of delay in evaluating safety data and can even prevent temporary IRB-imposed research holds during evaluation of a safety event.

Investigators are required by FDA regulations to communicate with IRBs about a number of clinical trial topics. Investigators must provide IRBs with all the necessary information on the study article to allow the IRB members to make an informed decision on approval or rejection of a study. IRBs must receive notification from the investigators of all changes to a study protocol. Investigators must also provide safety reports to the IRB as soon as the sponsor provides them to the investigators. These safety reports include information on different formulations or different strengths of the same product and may come from studies conducted both inside and outside the United States. Rather than rely on mail or fax, web-based email significantly speeds up communication, especially on a worldwide basis.

Communication between the sponsor and IRB occurs through the investigator. In current systems, communications between the study site personnel and the IRB is a paper-intensive process. The study coordinator and the investigator prepare information for the IRB to review and approve, including the protocol, the informed consent form and any advertisements that will be used for the study. An IRB must also notify the investigator in writing of its decision to approve, reject or request modification to a research project. The investigator must provide the sponsor with a copy of this correspondence, since the sponsor is also responsible for ensuring that studies are conducted in compliance with informed consent and IRB regulations. Internet-based communications save time so that study projects can get under way sooner and be managed more efficiently.

With electronic clinical trial systems, the site can provide electronic documents to the sponsor or CRO for evaluation. The site, the sponsor and the CRO can be networked to simultaneously acquire documentation and communications regarding the sites' qualifications for consideration as a study site. Qualification information and site personnel curriculum vitae [CVs] could be available online for review by the sponsor. The sample consent form can be provided to the study site online. Site personnel can customize the sample consent form to meet the IRB's requirements. It is already possible for the IRB to be connected via web-based EDC to the study personnel at the site and have access to the study data for safety reviews.

Often, sponsors will delay routine safety reviews until safety data are entered and cleaned sufficiently. This prevents unnecessary alarm or concern over data entry errors. The data management process involves a laborious serial process of double data entry, batch processing of automated safety checks, manual review of the safety checks and the data, release of data clarifications to site, re-entry of changed data and repeated cycles of the same. The result is that safety data are often not clean enough for review until weeks or months after the data are obtained. This can prevent important safety trends from being identified in a timely manner. An example of this might be the springtime surge in use of antihistamines as concomitant medications in a trial of a macrolide antibiotic. A seasonal increase in non-fatal arrhythmias might occur, but not be apparent to safety monitors until the fall. During this delay, tens or hundreds of patients could be exposed to a preventable risk. Electronic clinical trial systems allow for programming of edit checks that alert the study coordinator making the original entry of data to the system. In addition, manual review can occur daily allowing for early feedback. Data are more consistent and are available immediately for safety review in a cleaner form.

Referring Physicians

In many clinical trials a physician refers a patient to a clinical trial site to participate in a protocol. In these circumstances, referring physicians may lose touch with the progress of the patient, as patient data collected during the trial may not be easily available outside the site. As a result, physicians sometimes hesitate to enroll their patients in clinical trials. Once again, web clinical data management can make a difference. The referring physician can be given read-only access to the online clinical trial data through his or her web browser. In this way the referring physician would have up-to-date information on the patient without burdening the site with data transfer.

Medical Monitors

A medical monitor at a sponsor company has the responsibility for review of all adverse experiences, including serious adverse events during conduct of the study. In fulfilling this sponsor obligation, the medical monitor must review safety reports and look for trends in non-reported data, always considering the effect of the data on the continued investigation. EDC systems and Internet-based study communications can enhance the quality and efficiency of this role.

During the startup process, the medical monitor is a resource for establishing the expectations for safety review and assessments that will occur during the clinical study. The medical monitor presents the policies for data safety review at the investigator's meeting or at site initiation meetings. The electronic clinical trial system can be used as a resource for stating policies for the clinical study such as safety data collection and review requirements. The site personnel, sponsor personnel and all others could access and have this information available at all times. The medical monitor can be available by email to respond to questions that arise, and changes to study safety reporting policy can be posted on the web site. Details about reported serious adverse events can also be posted, allowing for review by investigators.

The medical monitor typically relies on the investigator and the investigative site staff to report serious adverse events. In obvious cases, the medical monitor will be notified immediately of an unexpected event. However, many sites fail to properly notify because they are busy, forget or are not sufficiently trained in the procedure. Inconsistency of site reporting of serious adverse events puts patients at risk and causes frustration for monitors.

Electronic clinical trial systems allow the medical monitor to review the data on a daily basis to identify potential serious adverse events. In addition, SAEs are often entered on CRFs, but the site hasn't informed the sponsor. It is easy to configure an electronic clinical trial system to send an email, fax or beeper notification to the appropriate individuals whenever an SAE is entered. The notification is automatic and immediate.

Once an SAE has been reported, the monitor can ensure the accuracy of data submitted to the FDA by reviewing individual subject data and comparing those records with the reports prepared by the investigator for submission to the sponsor. The medical monitor no longer has to rely on the site to fax or send in the CRFs. In addition, the medical monitor and data managers do not have to contend with data entered into a separate safety/AE system, which eventually must be reconciled with the clinical database—a typical scenario in companies today.

DSMB Oversight

In recent years, many clinical trials have included an independent data and safety monitoring board [DSMB]. This board consists of outside medical experts who periodically review the safety data from an ongoing clinical trial. These boards are independent of both the sponsor and institution and have the authority to stop a clinical trial immediately. The National Institutes of Health (NIH) now requires all NIH-funded or—conducted, multi-site clinical trials that entail potential risk to participants to establish DSMB oversight. The DSMB committees are required to share their summary study reports—such as adverse events—with designated IRBs. IRBs and DSMBs have the authority and mandate to review safety data. However, there is typically no mechanism for them to do so on a frequent basis. In paper-based clinical trials, members of these boards review data that have been received from the site and entered in the database—usually months or at least weeks old.

In a well-constructed electronic clinical trial data system, members of DSMBs can be given access to review patient data. This can be restricted to read-only access of just the data they are responsible for. This allows IRBs and DSMBs to look at an ongoing clinical trial without adding burden to the site. All they would need is a web browser and a password to enter the system. Now that it is technologically feasible to give access to clinical trial data, it can be argued that access should be an ethical imperative for safety monitoring boards.

Electronic clinical trial systems allow DSMB members to access currently available data. In some systems, status indicators show the data that are final, and raw data that have yet to be cleaned.

Patient Privacy

Patient privacy is an important aspect of clinical trials that can be affected by the power of eClinical trial systems. Consistent with Good Clinical Practices (GCP), pharmaceutical clinical research utilizes a process that removes patient identifiers from the data collected by the sponsor. Patients and subjects are referred to by study number, initials and date of birth. This should make it possible to protect privacy in many cases. It is noteworthy that these data, combined with other demographic data can often, with exhaustive investigative work, lead to the specific identification of a research subject. For this reason, it is essential that access to clinical trial data be heavily restricted, even if de-identified. In addition, investigators must have firm procedures in place to remove identification data wherever possible.

The FDA Electronic Records, Electronic Signatures Rule, 21 CFR 11, contains significant provisions for the security of electronic data collected in clinical trials (See Chapter 7.) The Health Insurance Portability and Accountability Act [HIPAA] was signed into law on August 21, 1996. The Final HIPAA Rule was promulgated on August 14, 2002, with a compliance date of April 14, 2003. The purpose of this broad-based law is to improve the efficiency and effectiveness of the healthcare system by encouraging the development of healthcare information systems using electronic data interchange [EDI] for health-related administrative and financial transactions. In addition, HIPAA seeks to establish the required use of national transaction standards while maintaining patient privacy when business and patient information is transmitted electronically between organizations.

The Administrative Simplification component of HIPAA requires Department of Health and Human Services [HHS] to develop standards and requirements for maintenance and transmission of health information that identifies individual patients. This component contains sections that will directly influence efforts to bring electronic solutions, such as EMRs, to the conduct of clinical trials. All vendors of EMR systems must conform to the standards in the Administrative Simplification component.

This component encompasses four standards:

1. Electronic transactions and code sets
2. Privacy of individually identifiable health information
3. Security to preserve patient confidentiality
4. Creation of unique health identifiers for patients, health plans, providers and employers

The fourth standard is one part of HIPAA that will directly affect clinical research. It addresses standards by which unique patient-identifying information can be transmitted electronically, possibly over the Internet. With growing concern over privacy issues, there is a great deal of interest in unique health identifiers for patients. Although they will use encryption, they will identify specific individuals. Investigative sites do not send names of study volunteers to sponsors or CROs, but there is still enough confidential information to require encryption. As of this writing, HHS has not yet published patient-identifying regulations. Regulations have been proposed for unique identifiers for national providers and employers, but they have not been finalized as of this writing.

In the European Union, the handling of clinical data is governed by the ICH Guideline for Good Clinical Practice (GCP). Directive 95/46/EC of the European Parliament and of the Council of 24 October 1995. An example of one of its limitations is found in Section 3, which prohibits the processing of personal data revealing racial or ethnic origin, political opinions, religious or philosophical beliefs, trade union membership and health status or sex life. Such processing becomes lawful if the subject gives explicit consent. Yet these types of data are relevant to clinical trials since different beliefs can lead to different practices that can affect health issues.

The interpretation of the EU Data Privacy Directives' impact on clinical trials is not yet certain. One of the major obstacles, transfer of data to the United States, is relieved by the development of U.S. Safe Harbor Principles. However, one major issue is the varied interpretations of the Directive by individual companies. This can cause considerable problems in implementing a multi-national clinical trial.

Keeping Data Private

When using electronic clinical trial systems for clinical data collection, patient privacy through data security must be considered. All clinical data passed between the web server and the user's web browser should move through a secure connection using encryption technology. The web application must be designed so that the browser connects securely to the web server using the secure socket layer (SSL) or other similar strong encryption technology. Through the use of these encryption technologies, the message is encrypted using a cryptographic formula called an encryption key. The resulting encrypted message can only be unscrambled, or decrypted, using a decryption key, which is mathematically related to it. With cryptography, any kind of digital information—text, data, voice, images—can be encrypted. These technologies make it virtually impossible to read clinical data during its transmission on the Internet.

The security of electronic clinical trial data goes beyond the actual transfer. At the local investigative site, an Internet-based clinical trial can be designed to leave no local data for tampering, "eavesdropping" or destruction. In cases where data are stored locally at the investigator site, physical security of the computer and a variety of operating procedures must be followed to restrict access to the data.

When properly designed and administered, an eClinical Trial can be the most secure form of data collection and management—far more secure and private than a paper-based clinical trial.

Conclusion

Safety review is a critical step in the conduct of clinical trials, both from an ethical perspective and in compliance with regulatory mandates. The current paper processes constrain the timely, proactive intercession by those responsible for assuring safety in clinical trials. The introduction of electronic clinical trials allows for more timely and even automatic notification and review of critical safety issues, allowing for greater patient protection. The clinical trials industry is reaching the point where research data can be made immediately available to IRBs and DSMBs so that they can provide a higher level of safety to patients. While Internet technology can be used for managing the safety of clinical trials, it must also be used judiciously to protect the privacy of patients and their health information.

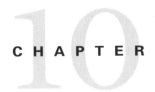

CHAPTER

Industry Data Standards: Ensuring the Success of Electronic Clinical Trial Implementations

Objectives

- Understand the importance of data standards and how they may affect the conduct of clinical trials.
- Identify two major standards organizations providing data models relevant to clinical trials.
- Describe the two major standard data models designed specifically for clinical trials and understand how and where they apply.
- List at least three benefits likely to be experienced by sites as a result of data standards.

While the new selection of electronic clinical trial (eCT) solutions are most promising, without standards for data exchange and storage, their benefits cannot be fully realized. Standards are necessary to harness the full potential of online clinical trial systems and the Internet. Standards enable easy data sharing among different solutions and easy communication of trial results to sponsors and regulatory agencies.

How important are data standards and compliance with them? So important that every new eCT technology purchase, every request for proposal (RFP), should include support for industry data standards as a prerequisite.

This chapter presents an overview of the standards that are pertinent to clinical sites. Some already are being applied behind the scenes to influence the way data are described on CRFs, and to control the transmission of data from systems already in use. Others will become more prominent in the future as new technologies emerge to dramatically improve the current clinical research process for sponsors and for sites.

The Value of Standards

Many aspects of our everyday life depend on standards. Credit and banking cards operate at a variety of automatic teller machines across the country and, in some cases, the world. Standards and codes are used to process financial transactions in a manner transparent to the end user. In medical practice, clinicians depend on standards to diagnose and treat medical conditions. In fact, the entire business of conducting clinical trials is governed by a mandated process standard that is collectively referred to as Good Clinical Practices, or GCP. An accepted fact of life in clinical trials is that, because there is no standard format for the data when they originally are recorded, the same data may be re-keyed or integrated into various databases numerous times. In addition to entering the data from CRFs into an operational database (twice) or transferring data from an EDC tool into the central database, the process also includes incorporating data from CROs or clinical laboratories. Then statistical programmers may have to make another round of transformations to analyze data from a single study or to combine data from multiple studies into an integrated summary database. Finally, if there's ever a need to reuse the data for some other indication, or for some other type of application, the data will probably have to be transformed again.

The pharmaceutical industry is so accustomed to this process that it seldom pauses to contemplate how inefficient and how primitive it really is. But most agree how much easier it could be—if only there were data standards.

Benefits of Industry Data Standards
In a new era, one that includes standards-based clinical research, sites will be far more comfortable collecting data because a significant portion of the data every study collects will contain the same essential items using the same questions, formats, structures and terms. And since this information is the same information that is recorded in internal systems (such as the site's patient database), a good portion of the information will be recorded only once at the source, and then be automatically and conveniently transferred using standard interfaces to other systems (such as clinical laboratories and sponsors) for other clinical trial purposes.

In a clinical trials world with information technology standards, sites will not have to wrestle with learning many different computer systems and processes used by different sponsors because most systems will have a similar look and feel. And even though the systems may be provided by different companies, they all will share a set of useful, familiar conventions, and they will all run on the same piece of hardware. Site personnel will not need as much retraining each time they do a new study. Everyone will focus more on information content, process, communication and people—rather than technology and problem-tracking. Every authorized individual will have rapid and trusted access to the information they need. In this world of standards, clinical research professionals will be able to do their jobs faster and more accurately, without unnecessary effort and frustration. Everybody involved in clinical trials will share in the benefits of standards.

These benefits for data interchange include:

- Increasing the familiarity with common data elements, thus reducing training requirements
- Improving data quality by reducing transcription errors and redundant data entry and by increasing site familiarity with data requirements
- Facilitating business processes and information exchange among biopharmaceutical companies, CROs, technology providers, clinical laboratories and regulatory agencies
- Reducing the time and cost associated with data interchange activities for clinical trials
- Facilitating regulatory reviews of submissions for market approvals
- Improving archiving methods for electronic clinical data so it will be available for future use or for compliance audits

History of Clinical Data Standards

Because clinical research is a scientific discipline, there has long been an inherent resistance to the application of standards by many of its participants. The fear is that such rigid structures would impede scientific freedom and slow down progress. In reality, science, by its very nature, is normally comfortable with the application of standard processes, methodologies, controls and formulae. Recently, resistance to data standards has slowly begun to erode thanks primarily to four important influencing factors:

- The consistent, ongoing tendency to streamline business processes with technology.
- The ongoing progress of the ICH and the FDA in defining an entire range of guidelines and standards relevant to clinical research.
- The cooperative efforts of individuals who believe strongly in the benefits of standards and have worked diligently to make them a reality in clinical research.
- The emergence of standards organizations dedicated to healthcare and clinical research

In truth, several relevant data standards are dealt with already in clinical research, as shown in Table 1. One of the most important recent standards efforts in the healthcare industry has been Health Level Seven (HL7),[1] an organization dedicated to developing standards for patient care and healthcare delivery. But, although HL7 has achieved broad acceptance within hospitals in the United States and has provided proven value in the healthcare industry for exchanging data among different types of related systems, it has not been viewed as being particularly suitable for use with clinical trials data (a presumption that is now beginning to change).

For sites that are currently using electronic medical record systems, HL7 should eventually offer many benefits because data that are already captured in other parts of the process theoretically can be transferred automatically to clinical trials electronic data capture systems. This would eliminate redundant data entry and transcription errors—and greatly reduce the workload at the site. Unfortunately, this is still purely theoretical for most clinical trials, and most sites still find themselves currently recording data once, twice, even three times on source documents, worksheets and CRFs.

Only recently have the efforts to define data standards progressed to the stage where they are a realistic near-term possibility. In clinical research, much of this progress is due to the work of the Clinical Data Interchange Standards Consortium (CDISC). CDISC was formed in 1997 as a grassroots effort of interested individuals and soon became a special interest advisory group of the Drug Information Association (DIA). Its vision is to establish worldwide industry standards to improve the process of acquiring and exchanging clinical trials information. Specifically, CDISC is an open, multidisciplinary organization committed to the development of worldwide industry standards to support the electronic acquisition, exchange, submission and archiving of clinical trials data and metadata for medical and biopharmaceutical product development. The CDISC mission is to lead the development of global, vendor-neutral, platform-independent standards to improve data quality and accelerate product development in our industry.[2]

In 2000, CDISC was established as a non-profit organization, and began to seriously ramp up its efforts to advance the standards movement. CDISC began pursuing its goals by initially defining a glossary of terms used in electronic clinical trials for drug development, while also beginning discussions on how to define a comprehensive data model for clinical trials. But when the latter effort stalled due to the great size of the task, CDISC shifted its attention to defining a model for improving the way data and metadata (information describing the structure and contents of a file or "data about data") are submitted as part of regulatory submissions. In effect, CDISC began to tackle the problem of data standards from the customer's viewpoint—the regulatory/FDA reviewer, who needs to make a product approval decision.

Table 1

A Sample of Data Standards Relevant to Clinical Development

Organization	Standard	Description
Health Level 7 (HL7)	HL7[3]	General messaging standard for exchange of general clinical orders, observations, claims data
College of American Pathologists (CAP)	Systemized Nomenclature of Human and Veterinary Medicine (SNOMED)[4,5]	Standardized medical dictionary of terms for diseases, clinical findings, etiologies, therapies, procedures, outcomes
American College of Radiology and National Electrical Manufacturers Association	DICOM[6]	Standard for exchange of medical images
LOINC Committee/ Regenstrief Institute	Logical Names, Identifiers and Codes (LOINC)[7]	Database of universal names and ID codes to facilitate the exchange and pooling of lab results for clinical care, outcomes management, research
National Cancer Institute (NCI)	Common Data Elements for Cancer Clinical Trials[8]	Object model and applications for conducting cancer research including common data elements, protocol development, eligibility
National Library of Medicine (NLM)	Unified Medical Language System (UMLS) Project[9]	Meta-thesaurus of vocabularies and knowledge sources

If standards could make it easier for regulatory reviewers to understand the contents of product marketing applications, CDISC reasoned, then reviewers could complete their reviews in less time and with less effort. And if product sponsors experienced such benefits and were encouraged by reviewers to conform, then standards would eventually be adopted throughout the clinical research life cycle. Thus, by agreeing on a core set of submission data standards (which became known as the CDISC submissions data model or SDM), industry would be defining standards potentially suitable for all clinical databases. This would have a ripple effect upstream to eventually benefit clinical research sites as well.

The strategy worked, because CDISC quickly resumed efforts on an operational data model (ODM) with renewed enthusiasm—a new model that would directly tackle the problem of moving data from any collection system to a clinical trial sponsor's central database. Figure 1 depicts the scope of the two initial CDISC models. Each of these primary models will be described briefly in the following sections.

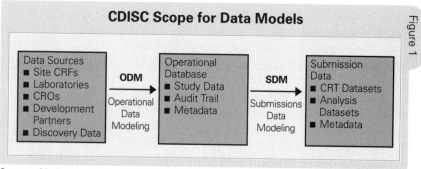

Source: CDISC Proprietary, March 2002

In 1999, the FDA published a series of guidelines related to electronic submissions.[10] These guidelines, which were created to advise pharmaceutical companies as they prepare to meet the FDA's stated future goal of receiving all regulatory submissions in electronic format, provided a great deal of information about submission documents. While they did specify that electronic data files would be required with submissions, they did not provide much detail on how best to prepare them.

With the encouragement and cooperation of several FDA participants, CDISC began to draft a metadata model for regulatory submissions. The CDISC submissions metadata model[11] provides a mechanism to improve the consistency and usefulness of data submissions for the benefit of FDA reviewers. Since the model is intended to address the organization and description of datasets accompanying electronic submissions (rather than data collection methods used by individual sites), many of its details are not directly relevant to this discussion. However, it is worth developing a very basic understanding of the model in order to see how it may affect the work of sites in the future.

The submissions model proposed common metadata standards, without rigid structures, to guide the organization of twelve common safety domains—particularly those data elements that would be common to almost any typical regulatory submission. While the initial model did not attempt to classify efficacy data, the metadata structures were designed to be relevant for any kind of submitted data, including statistical analysis datasets. The CDISC model focuses on metadata. Some of the metadata describes the organization and content of the individual dataset files; the remainder discusses the data variables themselves.

By listing the key data domains and their data elements, and providing a simple set of metadata characteristics about them, the CDISC model enables the FDA to fit each new submission into a common frame of reference. This helps them to better understand the content of each submission without substantial retraining or reorientation.

Within the SDM there are two variable-level metadata attributes that are most relevant to sites. The variable label is intended to clearly identify the contents of a variable. Ideally, this label should appear on the CRF or data collection tool and wherever the variable is used in tables and reports. The codes/formats attribute describes any codes or formats that are used for this field. The model encourages sponsors to decode the field with self-evident values, so they can be clearly understood by the reviewer (and originally by the sites). Over time, the CDISC group that developed the models has converged upon a number of standard conventions for use with data that should eventually be adopted by all. The end result will be a more standardized representation of data to be collected by sites, regardless of the company sponsoring the study, and less divergence between different data representations used in CRFs, eCRFs or data collection tools by different sponsors.

Another component of the metadata models that is relevant to sites is the concept of core variables. CDISC defines a core variable as one that normally should be present in all studies. While any individual study may require newly created variables that are only of relevance to that particular trial, each study should have the same set of core variables for data that describe patient identifiers, investigators, sex, race, visits, dates, times and other commonly used values.

As the SDM continues to evolve, it is being extended to additional types of data and also to the use of standard terminology used to record data. As data structures and vocabularies continue to become more standardized, sites will become more familiar with general data representations and require less training for each trial. This standardization also will reduce site vulnerability to misunderstandings and misinterpretations regarding clinical data.

The CDISC Operational Data Model

While the SDM describes how data are to be presented to FDA reviewers, it is not always directly applicable to the clinical data collected at investigative sites. As a result, sites must continually wrestle with the many different types of paper and eCRFs used to collect data and, in the case of EDC systems, may be required to use different types of systems for each individual trial. As more and more computer systems and eClinical trial technologies are developed and used by sponsors, the process of moving data from one system or company to another becomes more and more complicated. This is why the ODM was created.

The CDISC Operational Data Model was developed beginning in late 1999 by a small team of clinical system technologists, whose primary business involves clinical trials. The team began with two proposed models offered by two specific vendors. They then proceeded to create a new model based on the best features of each, plus other needs expressed in a list of requirements contributed by various stakeholders in the industry. The resulting model was written using the extensible markup language (XML), a language ideally suited for data interchange representation. XML was

developed by the World Wide Web Consortium (W3C)[12] as an open technical standard to exchange information between computer applications. XML
has been adopted in many industries as a foundation architecture for data
interchange, electronic commerce, and as a means of defining structured
documents. XML describes information[13] using simple text tags that can be
read by computers and people. As a matter of fact, XML allows for data to
describe itself to other computers, making data interfaces much simpler and
more reliable than in the past. For these reasons, XML was determined to be
the logical choice for the ODM.

Using an XML standard for interchange of clinical data could eliminate
the need to transcribe data manually from one system to another. The ability for sites to use their in-house scheduling and billing system to enroll or
examine a patient, and then have those same exact data available for reporting results in a clinical trial could yield enormous improvements in efficiency and quality. It would only be necessary to capture the clinical trial
data that were not previously available in the in-house systems.

Another advantage of XML is its ability to present data in a standard
structure that is independent of the device or application used to collect it.
With the power of XML, the same data file could be used to record a transaction even if the choice of input device varied. A traditional computer, a
palmtop computer, a wireless tablet, even a voice-activated computer or
interactive voice response system could all read or generate the same XML
file. This in itself could dramatically simplify the integration of technology
in clinical trials and make it possible to use whatever computer device is best
suited for each particular type of data being collected. Perhaps this would
even allow the site more say in the choice of which device to use for which
job.

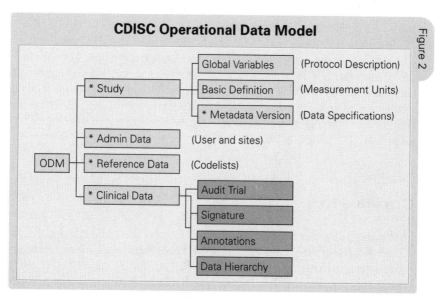

Figure 2

131

Finally, because XML includes both metadata and data, it forms an ideal data archiving mechanism. Even if a variety of different systems are used to collect data for different trials, the data can be stored in a similar way in a standard text file, and simple viewing tools can be provided to browse the data at any point in the future—no matter how much technology continues to evolve.

The CDISC ODM defines a standard XML representation for clinical study metadata and data. The major elements of the ODM XML model are illustrated in Figure 2.

The CDISC ODM has been tested and upgraded from Version 0.8 to 1.0 to 1.1 and is now being used for a variety of applications by many adopters within the industry.[14] With the CDISC ODM and XML, the practice of collecting data at investigative sites should eventually become a more familiar and seamless process, which will yield enormous benefits in terms of site productivity, ease of use and data consistency.

Further Progress on Clinical Data Standards

In 2001, CDISC and HL7 signed an agreement to have a formal association. The work toward harmonizing the standards of these two groups has been progressing within a technical committee formed to promote collaboration among representatives of FDA, HL7 and CDISC. In addition, LOINC codes are being recommended within appropriate areas of the CDISC models. These efforts signify a real interest in actually developing the means to facilitate the information connection between healthcare delivery and clinical trials—to make data sharing feasible.

In addition to the original SDM and ODM models, CDISC has also been actively developing associated models to address specific needs of the clinical laboratories (CDISC LAB model),[15] the statistical reviewers at regulatory agencies (ADaM model),[16] and other potential models. The newest focus is in the area of standards for protocol representation, which means that the ripple effect is finally making its way to the very beginning of the clinical trials process, the planning stage.

Conclusion

Data standardization is essential to improving the clinical trials process for all stakeholders—from sites and healthcare providers to sponsors and regulatory agencies. Through the efforts of CDISC, the FDA, HL7 and other organizations interested in this endeavor, data standards are finally becoming a reality in clinical research. The definition of common regulatory submission data standards can provide a fundamental basis for representing and reviewing the massive amounts of data that are collected during studies. The adoption of common XML data interchange standards such as those proposed by the CDISC operational data model will make data more readily available and more easily exchanged between healthcare providers and researchers. This should dramatically reduce cycle time for clinical development, which in turn will lead to increased availability of better, less costly therapies for the benefit of almost everyone.

By reducing the degree of variation that has been associated with clinical data in the past, standards will help technology vendors document basic assumptions, improve their understanding of clinical data and, as a result, deliver better, higher quality software products and components. In reality, open standards lead to increased interoperability, which eventually will make vendors concentrate more on improved functionality for the sites who use their product and improved quality. As clinical research standards continue to evolve, sites can expect to see greater uniformity in the look and feel of electronic clinical trial technologies and in the way the data are collected/entered into these systems.

Standards will be adopted eventually for many of the business processes involved in clinical trials, allowing sites to become more proficient in performing studies for different sponsors. This will eventually lead to a day when it no longer matters who provides the electronic clinical trial system—the sponsor or the site—since in the end all of the data will be delivered in the same way.

Endnotes

Chapter 8: Data Integrity

1. *Assuring Data Quality and Validity in Clinical Trials for Regulatory Decision Making.* Workshop Report, Institute of Medicine. National Academy Press: Washington, D.C., 1999.

2. McEntegart DJ et al. "Checks of case reports forms versus the database for efficacy variables when validation programs exist." *Drug Information Journal*, 33: 101-107, 1999.

Chapter 10: Industry Standards

1. Hiser, Robert E., Health Level Seven–Patient Management Standard. *In Electronic Communication Technologies A Practical Guide for Healthcare Manufacturers*, edited by Mervyn Mitchard, Denver: Interpharm Press, Inc.

2. CDISC Website, Concept Paper (*www.cdisc.org/pdf/CDISC-Concept.pdf*).

3. Health Level 7. (HL7) Available at: *http://www.hl7.org*. Last accessed: May 2001.

4. SNOMED: The Systematized Nomenclature of Human Medicine. Available at: *http://www.snomed.org*. Last Accessed: August 2000.

5. SNOMED: The Systematized Nomenclature of Human Medicine. Available at: *http://www.snomed.org.* Last Accessed: August 2000.

6. American College of Radiology (ACR)/National Electrical Manufacturers Association (NEMA). Digital Imaging and Communications in Medicine (DICOM). Available at: *http://www.nema.org/nema/medical/dicom.* Last accessed August 2000.

7. Logical Names, Identifiers and Codes (LOINC). Available at: *http://www.mcis.duke.edu/standards/termcode/loinc.html.* Last accessed: August 2000.

8. National Cancer Institute Common Data Elements for Cancer Clinical Trials. Available at: *http://cii.nci.nih.gov.* Last accessed: August 2000.

9. National Library of Medicine (NLM) Unified Medical Markup Language System (UMLS). Available at: *http://www.nlm.nih.gov/research/umls/umlsmain.html.* Last accessed: August 2000.

10. Guidance for Industry, Providing Regulatory Submissions in Electronic Format—General Considerations (IT-2, January, 1999). Available at *http://www.fda.gov/cder/guidelines.html.*
    Providing Regulatory Submissions in Electronic Format—NDAs (IT-3, January, 1999). Available at *http://www.fda.gov/cder/guidelines.htm.*
    Providing Regulatory Submissions in Electronic Format—Biologics Marketing Applications (November 1999). Available at *http://www.fda.gov/cder/guidelines.htm.*
    Example of an Electronic New Drug Application Submission (2/17/99). Available at *http://www.fda.gov/cder/guidelines.htm.*

11. CDISC Submissions Data Model; initial version proposed by Christiansen, David and Kubick, Wayne, CDISC Metadata Model for Electronic Submissions; Version 2.0 of Submissions Data Domain Models available at *http://www.cdisc.org/standards/index.html.*

12. World Wide Web Consortium (W3C) Extensible Markup Language (XML). Available at: *www.w3.org/XML/.* Last accessed: August 5, 1999.

13. Bosak, Jon and Bray, Tim. 1999. "XML and the Second Generation Web. Scientific American," Volume 280, Number 5, May, 1999: 89–93.

14. CDISC Operational Data Model *http://www.cdisc.org/standards /index.html.*

15. CDISC Clinical Laboratory Data Model under "standards." (*http://www.cdisc.org/standards/index.html.*)

16. CDISC Analysis Dataset Model Guidelines and Examples. (*http://www.cdisc.org/standards/index.html.*)

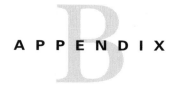

A P P E N D I X

Selected Reading

Bleicher, P. and Hauser, E. "Data Delivery During Crisis," *Applied Clinical Trials*, February 2002.

Bleicher, P. "Moving to Web-based Clinical Trials," *Global Outsourcing Review*, May 2002.

Borfitz, Deborah "Conspiring Forces Behind EDC Adoption," *CenterWatch*, February 2003.

Borfitz, Deborah "Building Momentum for Data Interchange Standards," *CenterWatch*, March 2003.

Bunn, Graham "Scaling Up ED," *Applied Clinical Trials 2002 EDC Supplement*, August 2002, 12-14.

CenterWatch Editorial, "A Unique EDC Adoption Obstacle in Europe," *CenterWatch*, March 2003.

Gambrill, Sara "The Unexpected Outcomes of 21 CFR 11 Compliance," *CenterWatch*, June 2002.

Henderson, Lisa "Will EDC Finally Catch On?" *CenterWatch*, September 1999.

Selected Reading

James, W.; Jones, D.; Ross, D. *The Machine That Changed the World*. Harper Perennial 1991.

Kubick, Wayne "The Elegant Machine: Applying Technology to Optimize Clinical Trials," *DIA Journal*, 1998, 861-869.

Kush, Rebecca "Data Standards for Clinical Development—Progress Update," *Applied Clinical Trials*, April 2002, 35-44.

Raymond, Steve "Interpretation of Regulatory Requirements by Technology Providers," *Applied Clinical Trials*, June 2002, 50-58.

Waegemann, C. Peter et al. (June 2002). Consensus Workshop on Health Information Capture and Report Generation Retrieved January 20, 2003 from www.medrecinst.com/media/document/summary.shtmml #cit1TOP.

Zisson, Stephen "A Market Receives EDC," *CenterWatch*, October 2001.

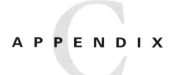
Glossary

Adverse Drug Reaction (ADR)

In the pre-approved clinical experience with a new medicinal product or its new usages, particularly as the therapeutic dose(s) may not be established: all noxious and unintended responses to a medicinal product related to any dose should be considered adverse drug reactions. The phrase *responses to a medicinal product* means that a causal relationship between a medicinal product and an adverse event is at least a reasonable possibility, i.e., the relationship cannot be ruled out.

Regarding marketed medicinal products: a response to a drug which is noxious and unintended and which occurs at doses normally used in man for prophylaxis, diagnosis, or therapy of diseases or for modification of physiological function [Note for Guidance on Good Clinical Practice (CPMP/ICH/135/95)]

(See the ICH Guideline for Clinical Safety Data Management: Definitions and Standards for Expedited Reporting)

Adverse Event (AE)

Any untoward medical occurrence in a patient or clinical investigation subject administered a pharmaceutical product and which does not necessarily have a causal relationship with this treatment. An adverse event (AE) can therefore be any unfavorable and unintended sign (including an abnormal laboratory finding), symptom, or disease temporally associated with the use of a medicinal (investigational) product, whether or not related to the medicinal (investigational) product function [Note for Guidance on Good Clinical Practice (CPMP/ICH/135/95)]

(See the ICH Guideline for Clinical Safety Data management: Definitions and Standards for Expedited Reporting.)

(Synonymous with *Adverse Experience*)

American National Standards Institute (ANSI)

Founded in 1918, ANSI itself does not develop standards. ANSI's roles include serving as the coordinator for U.S. voluntary standards efforts, acting as the approval body to recognize documents developed by other national organizations as American National Standards, acting as the U.S. representative in international and regional standards efforts, and serving as a clearinghouse for national and international standards development information. [HL7]

Application

Software designed to fill specific needs of a user; for example, software for navigation, payroll, or process control. [FDA-GL/IEEE]
(Synonym: *Application software*)

Application Service Provider (ASP)

Third-party entity that manages and distributes software-based services and solutions to customers across a wide area network from a central data center.

Audit trail

A secure, time stamped record that allows reconstruction of the course of events relating to the creation, modification and deletion of an electronic study record. [FDA Guidance on Computerized Systems Used in Clinical Trials]

Blinding

A procedure in which one or more parties involved in a clinical trial is kept unaware of the subject-specific treatment assignment(s). The purpose of blinding is to reduce bias error of data. Single blinding usually refers to the subject(s) being unaware, and double blinding usually refers to the subject(s), investigator(s), monitor and, in some cases, data analyst(s) being unaware of the treatment assignment(s). Open-label would mean that no one is blinded and the subject-specific study treatment is known to the investigator, sponsor and subjects. [SQA]

Case history

A record, in accordance with FDA 21 CFR 312.62b (specifying the requirement for investigator to prepare and maintain adequate and accurate case histories that record all observations and other data pertinent to the investigation on each individual administered the investigational drug [device or other therapy] or employed as a control in the investigation). [FDA]

NOTE: Case histories include the case report forms and supporting data, e.g., signed and dated informed consent forms, any medical records. Case histories shall document that patient informed consent was obtained prior to participation in the study.

Case report form (CRF)

A record of clinical study observations and other information designated in a clinical trial protocol to be completed for each study subject. [CDISC]

NOTE: In common usage, CRF can refer to either:

- a CRF page, which denotes a group of one or more data items that are linked together for purposes of collection and display.
- a CRF casebook, which denotes the entire group of CRF pages on which a set of clinical study observations and other information plan to be or to have been collected, or the information actually collected by completion of such CRF pages for a subject in a clinical study.

CRF (paper)

A CRF in which the data items on the CRF pages are linked by the physical properties of paper, for which data are captured manually and where any comments, notes, and signatures are also linked to those data items by writing or typescript on the paper CRF. [CDISC]

eCRF

An auditable electronic record designed to record information required by the clinical trial protocol to be reported to the sponsor on each trial subject (FDA Guidance on Computerized Systems Used in Clinical Trials); a CRF in which related data items and their associated comments, notes, and signatures are linked electronically. [CDISC]

NOTE: eCRFs may include special display elements, electronic edit checks and other special properties or functions and are used for both capture and display of the linked data.

Case report tabulations (CRT)

In a paper submission, listings of data that may be organized either by domain (type of data) or by patient. [CDISC]

CDISC

Acronym for Clinical Data Interchange Standards Consortium—an open, multidisciplinary, non-profit organization committed to the development of worldwide industry standards to support the electronic acquisition, exchange, submission and archiving of clinical trials data and metadata for medical and biopharmaceutical product development. [CDISC]

Clinical data
Data pertaining to the medical characteristics or status of a patient or subject. [CDISC]

Clinical efficacy (efficacy)
A relative concept referring to the ability of a therapy to elicit a beneficial clinical effect. [CDISC]

Clinical information
Clinical information refers to the data contained in the patient record. The data may include such things as problem lists, lab results, current medications, family history, etc. [HL7]

Clinical protocol
Document describing a clinical study and how it is to be conducted. A protocol includes the objectives of the study, the study design, a description of the test article(s) and dosage, the experimental procedure, handling of adverse reactions, how the results will be analyzed, and consent and clearance provisions. [SQA]

Clinical study
Synonym for Clinical trial.

Clinical trial
Any investigation in human subjects intended to discover or verify the clinical, pharmacological and/or other pharmacodynamic effects of an investigational product(s), and/or to identify any adverse reactions to an investigational product(s), and/or to study absorption, distribution, metabolism, and excretion of an investigational product(s) with the object of ascertaining its safety and/or effectiveness. [ICH]

NOTE: For the purposes of CDISC, this definition is extended to include medical devices and other investigational products for which clinical data are required for approval to market. [CDISC] (Synonyms: Clinical study, Clinical investigation)

Clinical trial data
See clinical trial information.

Clinical trial information
Data that are collected in the course of a clinical trial or relate to the integrity or administration of those data. [CDISC] (Synonym: *Clinical trial data*. See also *Data*.)

eClinical trial record
Any data collected electronically in support of a clinical trial, including, but not limited to, the eCRF data (e.g., medical history data, patient con-

tact information, IVRS data, electronic patient diary data, electronic health record data relevant to clinical trials, clinical laboratory data). [CDISC]

[NOTE: This term can be used to denote a "superset" of data, beyond what is required for the eCRF. An eClinical trial record typically includes electronic data that support documentation of complete clinical cases and case histories. Such electronic records may include, or be limited to, the protocol-specific clinical trial data such as electronic source documents.]

Control(s)

A well-controlled study permits a comparison of subjects treated with the investigational drug to a suitable control population, so that the effect of the investigational drug can be determined and distinguished from other influences, such as spontaneous change, placebo effects, concomitant therapy, or observer expectations. FDA regulations [21 CFR 312.126] cite several different kinds of controls that can be useful in particular circumstances:

- placebo-concurrent control
- dose comparison-concurrent control
- no-treatment-concurrent control
- active treatment-concurrent control, and
- historical control
- literature-based control [SQA]

Data

Representations of facts, concepts, or instructions in a manner suitable for communication, interpretation, or processing by humans or by automated means. [FDA-GL] (Synonym: *Information*)

Data element

(1) A named unit of data that, in some contexts, is considered indivisible and in other contexts may consist of data items. [ISO] (2) A named identifier of each of the entities and their attributes that are represented in a database. [FDA-GL]

Data entry

Input of data into a structured, computerized format using a human-computer interface (e.g., keyboard, pen-based tablet, voice recognition). [CDISC] (See also *electronic data capture*.)

Data integrity

The degree to which a collection of data is complete, consistent, and accurate. Integrity of data may be assessed in terms of whether they are attributable, legible, contemporaneous, original, and accurate. [derived from FDA-GL, FDA Guidance, IEEE]

Data interchange

The transfer of information between two or more parties. Data interchange is distinguished from data transfer in that the integrity of the contents of the data is maintained. [CDISC]

Data item

A named component of a data element; usually the smallest component. [ANSI] (See also *Data model*.)

Data model

Unambiguous, formally stated expression of items relationship, and structure of the data pertaining to a certain area or context of use. [CDISC]

NOTE: Unambiguous, as used above, means universally understood to have a single meaning.

Formally, as used above, means using agreed symbolic conventions to represent content so that communication of that content does not introduce ambiguity or otherwise lose the intended meaning.

Relationship, as used above, means characterized association between data item (e.g., ordinality, semantic).

Structure, as used above, means description of logical and physical organization: (permissible values, length, data type, etc.) (See also *CDISC Model-specific Terms*)

Data Safety Monitoring Board (DSMB)

A Data Safety Monitoring Board (DSMB) is a group of individuals with clinical expertise in the areas pertinent to the disease state and treatments being studied in controlled clinical trials. DSMBs typically also include a biostatistician who possesses a background and knowledge relevant to the conduct of clinical trials and analysis of clinical trial data and may also include an ethicist. As a group, the DSMB acts as an independent review/ advisory board whose primary mission is to measure and report on the continuing safety of current research subjects as well as subjects who have not yet enrolled. The DSMB accomplishes this through meeting on a regular basis and reviewing the accumulating data in an ongoing clinical trial. Through this process, the DSMB is also assessing the continuing validity and scientific merit of the trial.

Data security

The degree to which data are protected from exposure to accidental or malicious alteration or destruction. [derived from FDA-GL]

Data validation

(1) A process used to determine if data are inaccurate, incomplete, or unreasonable. The process may include format checks, completeness checks, check key tests, reasonableness checks and limit checks. [ISO] (2) The

checking of data for correctness or compliance with applicable standards, rules, and conventions. [FDA-GL]

Data verification
The process of ensuring that data at any point accurately represents the source data. [CDISC]

Domain
A category or type of data. The SDM uses the term to describe the core safety data domains: Demographics, Concomitant Medications, Exposure, Disposition, Adverse Events, Labs (includes Chemistry, Hematology, and Urinalysis), ECG, Vitals, Physical Examination, and History. [CDISC] Note: Would like to have an FDA definition, but couldn't find one.

Dosage form
The "delivery system" for a drug product, e.g., tablet, capsule, I.V. solution, topical cream, etc. [SQA]

Dosage
The amount of drug administered to a patient or test subject, either in a single administration or over the course of the clinical study. [CDISC]

Drug
(1) A substance recognized by an official pharmacopoeia or formulary, (2) a substance intended for use in the diagnosis, cure, mitigation, treatment, or prevention of disease, (3) a substance other than food intended to affect the structure or function of the body, (4) a substance intended for use as a component of a medicine but not a device or a component, part, or accessory of a device. [Food, Drug, & Cosmetic Act]

Drug development
The program for advancing a drug compound generally from the preclinical decision to recommend a single compound in a research program through its approval for marketing by the FDA and other regulatory agencies. [CDISC]

eCRT
CRTs provided in electronic format for eSubmissions (electronic regulatory submissions). [CDISC]

NOTE: According to current FDA guidance, eCRTs are datasets provided as SAS Transport files with accompanying documentation. They enable reviewers to analyze each dataset for each study. Each CRF domain should be provided as a single dataset, however additional datasets suitable for reproducing and confirming analyses may also be needed.

eClinical trial
A clinical trial in which primarily electronic processes are used to collect (acquire), access, exchange and archive data required for conduct, management, analysis and reporting of the trial. [CDISC] (synonyms: eClinical study; eClinical investigation)

Edit check
A validation rule electronically programmed to run on data. Note: edit checks commonly detect database data values outside of expected ranges or to identify missing data or dataset internal inconsistency. [CDISC]

Electronic Clinical Trial (eCT)
A clinical trial in which primarily electronic processes are used to plan, collect (acquire), access, exchange and archive data required for conduct, management, analysis and reporting of the trial. [CDISC]

Electronic data capture (EDC)
Collecting or acquiring data as a permanent electronic record with or without a human interface (e.g., using data collection systems or applications that are modem-based, web-based, optical mark/character recognition, or involve audio text, interactive voice response, graphical interfaces, clinical laboratory interfaces, or touch screens. [CDISC]

NOTE: "permanent" in the context of these definitions implies that any changes made to the electronic data are recorded via an audit trail.

Electronic record
Any combination of text, graphics, data, audio, pictorial, or any other information representation in digital form that is created, modified, maintained, archived, retrieved, or distributed by a computer system. [21 CFR, part 11]

Electronic signature
A computer data compilation of any symbol or series of symbols, executed, adopted, or authorized by an individual to be the legally binding equivalent of the individual's handwritten signature. [FDA Guidance on Computerized Systems Used in Clinical Trials]

Exclusion criteria
Items specified in a study protocol prohibiting subject participation in a clinical trial (e.g., medical restrictions, behavioral characteristics). [SQA]

NOTE: Exclusion and inclusion criteria define the study population.

Food and Drug Administration (FDA)
Within the Department of Health and Human Services. Enforces Food, Drug and Cosmetics Act and related federal public health laws. Grants IND, IDE, PMA and NDA approvals. (CenterWatch)

Good Clinical Practices (GCP)

A standard for the design, conduct, performance, monitoring, auditing, recording, analyses, and reporting of clinical trials that provides assurance that the data and reported results are credible and accurate, and that the rights, integrity, and confidentiality of trial subjects are protected. [SQA]

NOTE: for Guidance on Good Clinical Practice: CPMP/ICH/135/95; Declaration of Helsinki; USFDA 21 CFR Parts 50, 54, 56, and 312.

Health Level Seven (HL7)

An application protocol for electronic data exchange in healthcare environments. The HL7 protocol is a collection of standard formats which specify the implementation of interfaces between computer applications from different vendors. This communication protocol allows healthcare institutions to exchange key sets of data between different application systems. Flexibility is built into the protocol to allow compatibility for specialized data sets that have facility-specific needs. [HL7]

Health Insurance Portability and Accountability Act (HIPAA)

A law mandating that anyone belonging to a group health insurance plan must be allowed to purchase health insurance within an interval of time beginning when the previous coverage is lost. Establishes uniform, national standards for transactions, unique health identifiers, code sets for the data elements of the transactions, security of health information, and electronic signature.

Institute of Electrical and Electronics Engineers (IEEE)

An organization accredited by ANSI to submit its documents for approval as American National Standards; IEEE subcommittee P1073 develops standards for healthcare informatics: MEDIX (P1157) and MIB (P1073). [HL7]

Inclusion criteria

Essential characteristics the subject must have to be included in a clinical trial. [SQA]

NOTE: Exclusion and inclusion criteria define the study population.

Indication

Disease or condition for which a drug/device/therapy has been approved by the FDA or another regulatory agency. [CDISC]

Information

Synonym for *data.*

Informed consent

Process by which a subject voluntarily confirms his or her willingness to participate in a particular trial, after having been informed of all aspects of the trial that are relevant to the subject's decision to participate. Informed consent is documented by means of a written, signed, and dated Informed Consent Form. [SQA]

Informed consent form

Document approved by the Institutional Review Board/Ethics Review Committee (IRB/ERC) which describes to a potential subject the aims, methods, anticipated benefits, and potential hazards of an investigational study in a language he/she understands. [SQA]

Investigator

An individual who is qualified by training and experience (e.g., physician, dentist, clinical psychologist) to conduct a clinical study. He/she assumes direct responsibility for the welfare of subjects under his/her care, including the obligation to enroll subjects, to report adverse events, and to discontinue their treatment if there is real or anticipated danger. [SQA] (See also *principal investigator*.)

Institutional Review Board (IRB)

An independent group of professionals designated to review and approve the clinical protocol, informed consent forms, study advertisements, and patient brochures, to ensure that the study is safe and effective for human participation. It is also the IRB's responsibility to ensure that the study adheres to the FDA's regulations. (CenterWatch)

International Organization for Standardization (ISO)

A voluntary, non-treaty organization established in 1949 to promote international standards. Developers of the ISO Reference Model for Open Systems Interconnection (OSI Model), a standard approach to network design which introduces modularity by dividing the complex set of functions into more manageable self-contained, functional slices (layers). [HL7]

Interactive Voice Response Systems (IVRS)

An Interactive Voice Response System (IVRS), historically, is an interactive or touch-pad menu-driven system that takes the caller through a series of prompts. Callers then respond to questions by pressing buttons on the phone keypad. Most recently, with the convergence of handheld computers with cellular telephones, there has been substantial interest and early use of systems that involve simple EDC through a cell phone and/or a handheld computer with cellular access.

Labeling

Description of a drug and summary of use, safety, and effectiveness, as approved by the appropriate Regulatory Authority. [SQA]

Medical monitor
A sponsor representative who has medical authority for the evaluation of the safety aspects of a clinical trial. [SQA]

Metadata
Data that describe other data. [CDISC]

Monitoring
The act of overseeing a clinical trial, and of ensuring that it is conducted, documented, and reported in accordance with the protocol, standard operating procedures (SOP's), GCP, and the applicable regulatory requirement(s). [SQA] (See also *Medical Monitor.*)

Monitoring visit
A visit to a study site to review the progress of a clinical study and to ensure protocol adherence, accuracy of data, safety of subjects, and compliance with regulatory requirements and GCP guidelines. [SQA]

New Drug Application (NDA)
The compilation of all non-clinical, clinical, pharmacological, pharmacokinetic and stability information required about a drug by the FDA in order to approve the drug for marketing in the U.S. (CenterWatch)

Open-label
Study design in which drug given to subjects is known to both investigator and subjects. No placebo used. [SQA] (See *Blinding.*)

Operational Data Model (ODM)
A format for representing the study metadata, study data and administrative data associated with a clinical trial. It represents only the data that would be transferred among different software systems during a trial, or archived after a trial. It does not represent any information internal to a single system, for example, information about how the data would be stored in a particular database.

CDISC's intent is to make the format system-neutral, so the model is implemented in an XML DTD, which is an open, vendor-independent platform. [CDISC]

Order
A request for a service from one application to a second application. The second application may in some cases be the same, i.e., an application is allowed to place orders with itself. Usually orders are associated with a particular patient. [HL7]

Phase
Sequential evaluation of drugs/devices in humans. [CDISC]

Phase I clinical trials
Initial introduction of a new drug or biologic into humans at a stage when only animal and in vitro data are available. These studies are often referred to as "clinical pharmacology." These studies are primarily designed to determine the metabolism, pharmacological action and safety of the drug in humans. More specifically, Phase I studies help to determine a safe dosage range of the drug in humans, provides information of drug absorption, distribution, metabolism, and excretion (ADME), and possibly early evidence of effectiveness. Review of data from Phase I is important prior to proceeding to Phase II clinical development. Typical study characteristics for Phase I trials are:

- normal volunteers, patients occasionally
- 20-50 subjects
- close monitoring
- types of Phase I studies include:
- single dose
- ascending dose tolerance
- multiple dose
- seven (7) day ascending dose tolerance
- 28 day tolerance of highest dose [SQA]

Phase II clinical trials
First use of an investigational drug in humans to prevent or treat the disease for which it is intended. Close clinical monitoring is conducted on a relatively small number of subjects to determine the drug's short-term efficacy and its potential risks (safety). The characteristics for Phase II development include:

- Small, controlled studies
- Limited populations—100–200 subjects
- During Phase II it is essential to correlate blood levels with pharmacologic effects (i.e., pharmacodynamics and adverse events). As the results of Phase II trials, drugs with genuine potential are differentiated from those which are ineffective and/or not well tolerated. [SQA]

Phase III clinical trials
Expanded, controlled and uncontrolled clinical trials intended to gather additional evidence of efficacy for specific indications being studied and to better understand safety and drug related adverse effects. Phase III trials are usually large multi-center trials which collect substantial safety experience efficacy information and include the pivotal trials which serve the basis for drug approval. Phase III trials may also include specialized studies needed

for labeling (e.g., pediatric or elderly, comparative agents). Several hundred to several thousand patients may be included in the Phase III trials.

These studies are specifically designed to:

- verify effectiveness
- monitor effects from long term use
- establish labeling requirements
- determine overall risk/benefit
- model actual patient use [SQA]

Phase IV clinical trials

Marketing-oriented trials, conducted after the drug has been approved for marketing. Study design may extend the recommended duration of treatment or they may be primarily instructive in nature to help familiarize a larger number of practitioners with the drug's efficacy and side effects (seeding studies). [SQA]

Pivotal trials/studies

Adequate and well-controlled Phase II and III trials which provide the substantial evidence of effectiveness and safety upon which the drug is approved. Adequate and well-controlled trials possess the following characteristics:

- blinding
- randomization
- controls
- sufficient size [SQA]

Post-marketing surveillance

Clinical studies carried out by a company following market introduction to evaluate a new drug under conditions of actual medical practice. The studies may be initiated by the manufacturer to clarify why and how a new drug is used and determine whether the adverse experience profile established in controlled trials reflects the true properties of the drug. Such studies may also be required by a regulatory health authority as a condition for approval. [SQA]

Principal investigator

Investigator held primarily responsible (as indicated on FDA Form 1572, for example) for the clinical conduct of a study carried-out under his/her auspices. [SQA] (See also *Investigator*)

Protocol

A detailed plan that sets forth the objectives, study design, and methodology for a clinical trial. A study protocol must be approved by an IRB before investigational drugs may be administered to humans. (CenterWatch)

Protocol amendment
Written description of a change(s) to, or formal clarification of, a clinical protocol. [SQA]

Quality assurance
All those planned and systematic actions that are established to ensure that the trial is performed, and the data are generated, documented (recorded), and reported in compliance with GCP and the applicable regulatory requirement(s). [SQA]

Quality control
The operational techniques and activities undertaken within the quality assurance system to verify that the requirements for quality of the trial-related activities have been fulfilled. [SQA]

Randomization
The process of assigning trial subjects to treatment or control groups using an element of chance to determine the assignments in order to reduce bias. [SQA]

Raw data
Researcher's records of patients, such as patient charts, hospital records, X-rays, and attending physician's notes. These records may or may not accompany an application to a Regulatory Authority, but must be kept in the researcher's file. [SQA]

Regulatory Agency
Many geopolitical entities have established agencies/authority responsible for regulating products used in healthcare. The agencies are collectively referred to as regulatory agencies. [HL7]

Screen/Screening
(1) The process by which substances are evaluated in a battery of tests or assays (screens) designed to detect a specific biological property or activity. It can be conducted on a random basis in which substances are tested without any pre-selection criteria or on a targeted basis in which information on a substance with known activity and structure is used as a basis for selecting other similar substances on which to run the battery of tests. (2) Determining the suitability of an investigatory site and personnel to participate in a clinical trial. [SQA]

Serious adverse event (SAE)
Any adverse experience occurring at any dose that results in any of the following outcomes: death, a life-threatening adverse experience, inpatient hospitalization or prolongation of existing hospitalization, a persistent or significant disability/incapacity, or a congenital anomaly/birth defect.

Important medical events that may not result in death, be life threatening, or require hospitalization may be considered a serious adverse drug experience when, based upon appropriate medical judgment, they may jeopardize the patient or subject and may require medical or surgical intervention to prevent one. [ICH]

Software
Computer programs pertaining to the operation of a system. [derived from FDA-GL/ANSI]

Society of Quality Assurance (SQA)
Professional organization founded to promote the quality assurance profession through the discussion and exchange of ideas and the promulgation and continued advancement of high professional standards.

Source data
All information in original records, certified records, and certified copies of original records of clinical findings; observations; or other activities in a clinical trial necessary for the reconstruction and evaluation of the trial. Source data are contained in source documents (original records or certified copies). [ICH]

eSource data (electronic Source data)
Source data (per FDA/ICH definition) captured initially into a permanent electronic record. [CDISC]
NOTE: "permanent" in the context of these definitions implies that any changes made to the electronic data are recorded via an audit trail.

Source documents
Original documents, data, and records (e.g., hospital records, clinical and office charts, laboratory notes, memoranda, subject's diaries or evaluation checklists, pharmacy dispensing records, recorded data from automated instruments, copies or transcriptions certified after verification as being accurate copies, microfiches, photographic negatives, microfilm or magnetic media, X-rays, subject files, and records kept at the pharmacy, at the laboratories and at medico-technical departments involved in the clinical trial). [ICH]

Sponsor
A company or individual which plans and initiates clinical drug studies for new products. Usually, the sponsor is the party that has submitted the Investigational New Drug Application (IND/IDD) to the Regulatory Authority to allow testing in humans. [SQA]

Sponsor-Investigator

Individual who both initiates and conducts, alone or with others, a clinical trial, and under whose immediate direction the investigational product is administered to, dispensed to, or used by a subject. The term does not include any person other than an individual (e.g., it does not include a corporation or an agency). The obligations of a sponsor-investigator include both those of a sponsor and those of an investigator. [SQA]

Standard Operating Procedures (SOPs)

Written instructions describing operations to be performed and methods employed. [SQA]

Study coordinator

Member of site personnel. Responsible for the day-to-day running of the clinical trial. [CDISC]

Subject

Human participant in a clinical trial. [SQA]

Sub-investigator

Individual member of the clinical trial team designated and supervised by the investigator at a trial site to perform critical trial related procedures and/or to make important trial related decisions (e.g., associates, residents, research fellows). For studies conducted in the US, or from which data are to be submitted to the FDA, sub-investigators must be included on the FDA Form 1572. [SQA]

Submissions Data Model (SDM)

The CDISC Submissions Data Model has been prepared by the CDISC Submissions Data Standards (SDS) team to guide the organization, content, and form of submission datasets for the 12 safety-related domains listed in the FDA guidance documents. In the future, additional models will be provided for common analysis formats and to describe other types of data such as pharmacokinetics and pharmacodynamics, as well as efficacy data for certain therapeutic areas. [CDISC]

System

People, machines, software, applications and/or methods organized to accomplish a set of specific functions or objectives. [derived from FDA-GL/ANSI]

Technology provider

Person, company or other entity who develops, produces and sells software applications and/or hardware for use in conducting clinical trials and/or in analyzing clinical trial data and or submitting clinical trial information for regulatory approval. [CDISC] (Synonym: *Vendor*).

Transcription

A process of transforming dictated or otherwise documented information into an electronic format. [HL7]

Unexpected adverse experience

Any adverse drug experience that is not listed in the current labeling or Investigator's Brochure for the drug product or for which the incidence experienced by clinical trial subjects is notably greater than that included in the labeling or Investigator's Brochure. This includes events that may be symptomatically and pathophysiologically related to an event listed in the labeling, but differ from the event because of greater severity, specificity, or frequency. For example, under this definition, hepatic necrosis would be unexpected (by virtue of greater severity) if the labeling only referred to elevated hepatic enzymes or hepatitis. Similarly, cerebral thromboembolism and cerebral vasculitis would be unexpected (by virtue of greater specificity) if the labeling only listed cerebral vascular accidents. "Unexpected," as used in this definition, refers to an adverse drug experience that has not been previously observed (i.e., included in the labeling) rather than from the perspective of such experience not being anticipated from the pharmacological properties of the pharmaceutical product.) [SQA]

World-Wide Web Consortium (W3C)

Develops interoperable technologies (specifications, guidelines, software, and tools) to lead the Web to its full potential. W3C is a forum for information, commerce, communication, and collective understanding.

XML

An acronym for eXtensible Markup Language. XML is a computer programming language that supports the definition and representation of sophisticated data models in a consistent text-based (ASCII) format—one that can be processed conveniently by a growing set of third-party tools. XML is gaining wide acceptance as a data interchange framework in other industries and is beginning to be utilized by several vendors of clinical trials software products. [CDISC]

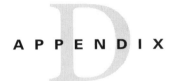

APPENDIX D

Traceability Matrix

Component of the Rule	Compliance Documentation
11.10 Controls for Closed Systems Persons who use closed systems to create, modify, maintain, or transmit electronic records shall employ procedures and controls designed to ensure the authenticity, integrity, and, when appropriate, the confidentiality of electronic records, and to ensure that the signer cannot readily repudiate the signed record as not genuine. Such procedures and controls shall include the following:	SOPs, test documents, handwritten agreements, etc. See below.
(a) Validation of systems to ensure accuracy, reliability, consistent intended performance, and the ability to discern invalid or altered records.	Trial validation
(b) The ability to generate accurate and complete copies of records in both human readable and electronic form suitable for inspection, review, and copying by the agency. Persons should contact the agency	A test result

Component of the Rule	Compliance Documentation
if there are any questions regarding the ability of the agency to perform such review and copying of the electronic records.	
(c) Protection of records to enable their accurate and ready retrieval throughout the records retention period.	Trial system security SOP Trial system backup & restore SOP Trial system disaster recovery SOP Trial archive SOP
(d) Limiting system access to authorized individuals.	Trial system security
(e) Use of secure, computer-generated, time-stamped audit trails to independently record the date and time of operator entries and actions that create, modify, or delete electronic records. Record changes shall not obscure previously recorded information. Such audit trail documentation shall be retained for a period at least as long as that required for the subject electronic records and shall be available for agency review and copying.	Audit trail tests Computer generated copy
(f) Use of operational system checks to enforce permitted sequencing of steps and events, as appropriate.	As per protocol
(g) Use of authorization checks to ensure that only authorized individuals can use the system, electronically sign a record, access the operation or computer system input or output device, alter a record, or perform the operation at hand.	Specify authorization checks Specify identity docs

Component of the Rule	Compliance Documentation
(h) Use of device (e.g., terminal) checks to determine, as appropriate, the validity of the source of data input or operational instruction.	Device qualification
(i) Determination that persons who develop, maintain, or use electronic record/electronic signature systems have the education, training, and experience to perform their assigned tasks.	Training records SOP Training doc
(j) The establishment of, and adherence to, written policies that hold individuals accountable and responsible for actions initiated under their electronic signatures, in order to deter record and signature falsification.	Electronic signature agreement
(k) Use of appropriate controls over systems documentation including: (1) Adequate controls over the distribution of, access to, and use of documentation for system operation and maintenance. (2) Revision and change control procedures to maintain an audit trail that documents time-sequenced development and modification of systems documentation.	Document controls System documents Site training manuals
11.30 Controls for Open Systems Persons who use open systems to create, modify, maintain, or transmit electronic records shall employ procedures and controls designed to ensure the authenticity, integrity, and, as appropriate, the confidentiality of electronic records from the point of their creation to the point of their receipt. Such procedures and controls shall include those identified in Sec. 11.10, as appropriate, and additional measures such as document encryption and use of appropriate digital signature standards to ensure, as necessary under the circumstances, record authenticity, integrity, and confidentiality.	Encryption documentation Security challenge testing documents Security audits

Component of the Rule	Compliance Documentation
11.50 Signature manifestations. (a) Signed electronic records shall contain information associated with the signing that clearly indicates all of the following:	
(1) The printed name of the signer	
(2) The date and time when the signature was executed	Time stamp present and documented tests for accuracy
(3) The meaning (such as review, approval, responsibility, or authorship) associated with the signature.	Affidavit available
(b) The items identified in paragraphs (a)(1), (a)(2), and (a)(3) of this section shall be subject to the same controls as for electronic records and shall be included as part of any human readable form of the electronic record (such as electronic display or printout).	Check printouts
11.70 Signature/record linking. Electronic signatures and handwritten signatures executed to electronic records shall be linked to their respective electronic records to ensure that the signatures cannot be excised, copied, or otherwise transferred to falsify an electronic record by ordinary means.	Validation docs

C--Electronic Signatures

11.100 General requirements.

(a) Each electronic signature shall be unique to one individual and shall not be reused by, or reassigned to, anyone else.	Process and technology check
(b) Before an organization establishes, assigns, certifies, or otherwise sanctions an individual's electronic signatures, or any ele-	Identity verification procedures documented

Component of the Rule	Compliance Documentation

ment of such electronic signature, the organization shall verify the identity of the individual.

(c) Persons using electronic signatures shall, prior to or at the time of such use, certify to the agency that the electronic signatures in their system, used on or after August 20, 1997, are intended to be the legally binding equivalent of traditional handwritten signatures.

Policy document

Docs from each user

(1) The certification shall be submitted in paper form and signed with a traditional handwritten signature, to the Office of Regional Operations (HFC-100), 5600 Fishers Lane, Rockville, MD 20857.

Letter to Agency

(2) Persons using electronic signatures shall, upon agency request, provide additional certification or testimony that a specific electronic signature is the legally binding equivalent of the signer's handwritten signature.

Capability to recover doc from each user

11.200 Electronic signature components and controls.

(a) Electronic signatures that are not based upon biometrics shall:

(1) Employ at least two distinct identification components such as an identification code and password.

Login and password

(i) When an individual executes a series of signings during a single, continuous period of controlled system access, the first signing shall be executed using all electronic signature components; subsequent signings shall be executed using at least one electronic signature component

System validation docs

Component of the Rule	Compliance Documentation
that is only executable by, and designed to be used only by, the individual.	
(ii) When an individual executes one or more signings not performed during a single, continuous period of controlled system access, each signing shall be executed using all of the electronic signature components.	Timeouts, repeat login
(2) Be used only by their genuine owners.	Process definition and tech checks
(3) Be administered and executed to ensure that attempted use of an individual's electronic signature by anyone other than its genuine owner requires collaboration of two or more individuals.	Process definitions and tech checks
(b) Electronic signatures based upon biometrics shall be designed to ensure that they cannot be used by anyone other than their genuine owners.	Validation testing of biometric technology
11.300 Controls for identification codes/passwords. Persons who use electronic signatures based upon use of identification codes in combination with passwords shall employ controls to ensure their security and integrity. Such controls shall include:	Will electronic signatures be used?
(a) Maintaining the uniqueness of each combined identification code and password, such that no two individuals have the same combination of identification code and password.	System validation docs
(b) Ensuring that identification code and password issuances are periodically checked, recalled, or revised (e.g., to cover such events as password aging).	System design, system validation docs

Component of the Rule	**Compliance Documentation**
(c) Following loss management procedures to electronically invalidate lost, stolen, missing, or otherwise potentially compromised tokens, cards, and other devices that bear or generate identification code or password information, and to issue temporary or permanent replacements using suitable, rigorous controls.	System validation tests for invalidation; tests for password process
(d) Use of transaction safeguards to prevent unauthorized use of passwords and/or identification codes, and to detect and report in an immediate and urgent manner any attempts at their unauthorized use to the system security unit, and, as appropriate, to organizational management.	Process documents SOPs Evidence of use
(e) Initial and periodic testing of devices, such as tokens and cards, that bear or generate identification code or password information to ensure that they function properly and have not been altered in an unauthorized manner.	SOPs and documentation of testing

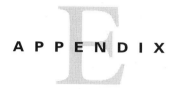

APPENDIX E

21 CFR Part 11

Electronic Records; Electronic Signatures

Subpart A—General Provisions

11.1   Scope.
11.2   Implementation.
11.3   Definitions.

Subpart B—Electronic Records

11.10   Controls for closed systems.
11.30   Controls for open systems.
11.50   Signature manifestations.
11.70   Signature/record linking.

Subpart C—Electronic Signatures

11.100   General requirements.
11.200   Electronic signature components and controls.
11.300   Controls for identification codes/passwords.

Authority: 21 U.S.C. 321-393; 42 U.S.C. 262.

Source: 62 FR 13464, Mar. 20, 1997, unless otherwise noted.

Subpart A — General Provisions

§11.1 Scope.

(a) The regulations in this part set forth the criteria under which the agency considers electronic records, electronic signatures, and handwritten signatures executed to electronic records to be trustworthy, reliable, and generally equivalent to paper records and handwritten signatures executed on paper.

(b) This part applies to records in electronic form that are created, modified, maintained, archived, retrieved, or transmitted, under any records requirements set forth in agency regulations. This part also applies to electronic records submitted to the agency under requirements of the Federal Food, Drug, and Cosmetic Act and the Public Health Service Act, even if such records are not specifically identified in agency regulations. However, this part does not apply to paper records that are, or have been, transmitted by electronic means.

(c) Where electronic signatures and their associated electronic records meet the requirements of this part, the agency will consider the electronic signatures to be equivalent to full handwritten signatures, initials, and other general signings as required by agency regulations, unless specifically excepted by regulation(s) effective on or after August 20, 1997.

(d) Electronic records that meet the requirements of this part may be used in lieu of paper records, in accordance with §11.2, unless paper records are specifically required.

(e) Computer systems (including hardware and software), controls, and attendant documentation maintained under this part shall be readily available for, and subject to, FDA inspection.

§11.2 Implementation.

(a) For records required to be maintained but not submitted to the agency, persons may use electronic records in lieu of paper records or electronic signatures in lieu of traditional signatures, in whole or in part, provided that the requirements of this part are met.

(b) For records submitted to the agency, persons may use electronic records in lieu of paper records or electronic signatures in lieu of traditional signatures, in whole or in part, provided that:

(1) The requirements of this part are met; and

(2) The document or parts of a document to be submitted have been identified in public docket No. 92S-0251 as being the type of submission the agency accepts in electronic form. This docket will identify specifically what types of documents or parts of documents are acceptable for submission in electronic form without paper records and the agency receiving unit(s) (e.g., specific center, office, division, branch) to which such submissions may be made. Documents to agency receiving unit(s) not specified in the public docket will not be considered as official if they are submitted in electronic form; paper forms of such documents will be considered as official and must accompany any electronic records. Persons are expected to consult with the intended agency receiving unit for details on how (e.g., method of transmission, media, file formats, and technical protocols) and whether to proceed with the electronic submission.

§11.3 Definitions.

(a) The definitions and interpretations of terms contained in section 201 of the act apply to those terms when used in this part.

(b) The following definitions of terms also apply to this part:

(1 *Act* means the Federal Food, Drug, and Cosmetic Act (secs. 201-903 (21 U.S.C. 321-393)).

(2 *Agency* means the Food and Drug Administration.

(3) *Biometrics* means a method of verifying an individual's identity based on measurement of the individual's physical feature(s) or repeatable action(s) where those features and/or actions are both unique to that individual and measurable.

(4) *Closed system* means an environment in which system access is controlled by persons who are responsible for the content of electronic records that are on the system.

(5) *Digital signature* means an electronic signature based upon cryptographic methods of originator authentication, computed by using a set of rules and a set of parameters such that the identity of the signer and the integrity of the data can be verified.

(6) *Electronic record* means any combination of text, graphics, data, audio, pictorial, or other information representation in digital form that is created, modified, maintained, archived, retrieved, or distributed by a computer system.

(7) *Electronic signature* means a computer data compilation of any symbol or series of symbols executed, adopted, or authorized by an individual to be the legally binding equivalent of the individual's handwritten signature.

(8) *Handwritten signature* means the scripted name or legal mark of an individual handwritten by that individual and executed or adopted with the present intention to authenticate a writing in a permanent form. The act of signing with a writing or marking instrument such as a pen or stylus is preserved. The scripted name or legal mark, while conventionally applied to paper, may also be applied to other devices that capture the name or mark.

(9) *Open system* means an environment in which system access is not controlled by persons who are responsible for the content of electronic records that are on the system.

Subpart B — Electronic Records

§11.10 Controls for closed systems.
Persons who use closed systems to create, modify, maintain, or transmit electronic records shall employ procedures and controls designed to ensure the authenticity, integrity, and, when appropriate, the confidentiality of electronic records, and to ensure that the signer cannot readily repudiate the signed record as not genuine. Such procedures and controls shall include the following:

(a) Validation of systems to ensure accuracy, reliability, consistent intended performance, and the ability to discern invalid or altered records.

(b) The ability to generate accurate and complete copies of records in both human readable and electronic form suitable for inspection, review, and copying by the agency. Persons should contact the agency if there are any questions regarding the ability of the agency to perform such review and copying of the electronic records.

(c) Protection of records to enable their accurate and ready retrieval throughout the records retention period.

(d) Limiting system access to authorized individuals.

(e) Use of secure, computer-generated, time-stamped audit trails to independently record the date and time of operator entries and actions that create, modify, or delete electronic records. Record changes shall not obscure previously recorded information. Such audit trail documentation shall be retained for a period at least as long as that required for the subject electronic records and shall be available for agency review and copying.

(f) Use of operational system checks to enforce permitted sequencing of steps and events, as appropriate.

(g) Use of authority checks to ensure that only authorized individuals can use the system, electronically sign a record, access the operation or computer system input or output device, alter a record, or perform the operation at hand.

(h) Use of device (e.g., terminal) checks to determine, as appropriate, the validity of the source of data input or operational instruction.

(i) Determination that persons who develop, maintain, or use electronic record/electronic signature systems have the education, training, and experience to perform their assigned tasks.

(j) The establishment of, and adherence to, written policies that hold individuals accountable and responsible for actions initiated under their electronic signatures, in order to deter record and signature falsification.

(k) Use of appropriate controls over systems documentation including:

(1) Adequate controls over the distribution of, access to, and use of documentation for system operation and maintenance.

(2) Revision and change control procedures to maintain an audit trail that documents time-sequenced development and modification of systems documentation.

§11.30 Controls for open systems.
Persons who use open systems to create, modify, maintain, or transmit electronic records shall employ procedures and controls designed to ensure the authenticity, integrity, and, as appropriate, the confidentiality of electronic records from the point of their creation to the point of their receipt. Such procedures and controls shall include those identified in §11.10, as appropriate, and additional measures such as document encryption and use of appropriate digital signature standards to ensure, as necessary under the circumstances, record authenticity, integrity, and confidentiality.

§11.50 Signature manifestations.

(a) Signed electronic records shall contain information associated with the signing that clearly indicates all of the following:

(1) The printed name of the signer;

(2) The date and time when the signature was executed; and

(3) The meaning (such as review, approval, responsibility, or authorship) associated with the signature.

(b) The items identified in paragraphs (a)(1), (a)(2), and (a)(3) of this section shall be subject to the same controls as for electronic records and shall be included as part of any human readable form of the electronic record (such as electronic display or printout).

§11.70 Signature/record linking.

Electronic signatures and handwritten signatures executed to electronic records shall be linked to their respective electronic records to ensure that the signatures cannot be excised, copied, or otherwise transferred to falsify an electronic record by ordinary means.

Subpart C — Electronic Signatures

§11.100 General requirements.

(a) Each electronic signature shall be unique to one individual and shall not be reused by, or reassigned to, anyone else.

(b) Before an organization establishes, assigns, certifies, or otherwise sanctions an individual's electronic signature, or any element of such electronic signature, the organization shall verify the identity of the individual.

(c) Persons using electronic signatures shall, prior to or at the time of such use, certify to the agency that the electronic signatures in their system, used on or after August 20, 1997, are intended to be the legally binding equivalent of traditional handwritten signatures.

(1) The certification shall be submitted in paper form and signed with a traditional handwritten signature, to the Office of Regional Operations (HFC-100), 5600 Fishers Lane, Rockville, MD 20857.

(2) Persons using electronic signatures shall, upon agency request, provide additional certification or testimony that a specific electronic signature is the legally binding equivalent of the signer's handwritten signature.

§11.200 Electronic signature components and controls.

(a) Electronic signatures that are not based upon biometrics shall:

(1) Employ at least two distinct identification components such as an identification code and password.

    (i) When an individual executes a series of signings during a single, continuous period of controlled system access, the first signing shall be executed using all electronic signature components; subsequent signings shall be executed using at least one electronic signature component that is only executable by, and designed to be used only by, the individual.

    (ii) When an individual executes one or more signings not performed during a single, continuous period of controlled system access, each signing shall be executed using all of the electronic signature components.

(2) Be used only by their genuine owners; and

(3) Be administered and executed to ensure that attempted use of an individual's electronic signature by anyone other than its genuine owner requires collaboration of two or more individuals.

(b) Electronic signatures based upon biometrics shall be designed to ensure that they cannot be used by anyone other than their genuine owners.

§11.300 Controls for identification codes/passwords.

Persons who use electronic signatures based upon use of identification codes in combination with passwords shall employ controls to ensure their security and integrity. Such controls shall include:

(a) Maintaining the uniqueness of each combined identification code and password, such that no two individuals have the same combination of identification code and password.

(b) Ensuring that identification code and password issuances are periodically checked, recalled, or revised (e.g., to cover such events as password aging).

(c) Following loss management procedures to electronically deauthorize lost, stolen, missing, or otherwise potentially compromised tokens, cards, and other devices that bear or generate identification code or password information, and to issue temporary or permanent replacements using suitable, rigorous controls.

(d) Use of transaction safeguards to prevent unauthorized use of passwords and/or identification codes, and to detect and report in an immediate and urgent manner any attempts at their unauthorized use to the system security unit, and, as appropriate, to organizational management.

(e) Initial and periodic testing of devices, such as tokens or cards, that bear or generate identification code or password information to ensure that they function properly and have not been altered in an unauthorized manner.

F
A P P E N D I X

Guidance for Industry: Computerized Systems Used in Clinical Trials [CSUCT]

I. Introduction

This document addresses issues pertaining to computerized systems used to create, modify, maintain, archive, retrieve, or transmit clinical data intended for submission to the Food and Drug Administration (FDA). These data form the basis for the Agency's decisions regarding the safety and efficacy of new human and animal drugs, biologics, medical devices, and certain food and color additives. As such, these data have broad public health significance and must be of the highest quality and integrity.

FDA established the Bioresearch Monitoring (BIMO) Program of inspections and audits to monitor the conduct and reporting of clinical trials to ensure that data from these trials meet the highest standards of quality and integrity and conform to FDA's regulations. FDA's acceptance of data from clinical trials for decision-making purposes is dependent upon its ability to verify the quality and integrity of such data during its onsite inspections and audits. To be acceptable the data should meet certain fundamental elements of quality whether collected or recorded electronically or on paper. Data should be attributable, original, accurate, contemporaneous, and legible. For example, attributable data can be traced to individuals responsible for observing and recording the data. In an automated system, attributability could be achieved by a computer system designed to identify individuals responsible for any input.

This guidance addresses how these elements of data quality might be satisfied where computerized systems are being used to create, modify, maintain, archive, retrieve, or transmit clinical data. Although the primary focus of this guidance is on computerized systems used at clinical sites to collect data, the principles set forth may also be appropriate for computerized systems at contract research organizations, data management centers, and sponsors. Persons using the data from computerized systems should have confidence that the data are no less reliable than data in paper form.

Computerized medical devices, diagnostic laboratory instruments and instruments in analytical laboratories that are used in clinical trials are not the focus of this guidance. This guidance does not address electronic submissions or methods of their transmission to the Agency.

This guidance document reflects long-standing regulations covering clinical trial records. It also addresses requirements of the Electronic Records/Electronic Signatures rule (21 CFR part 11).

The principles in this guidance may be applied where source documents are created (1) in hardcopy and later entered into a computerized system, (2) by direct entry by a human into a computerized system, and (3) automatically by a computerized system.

II. Definitions

Audit Trail means, for the purposes of this guidance, a secure, computer generated, time-stamped electronic record that allows reconstruction of the course of events relating to the creation, modification, and deletion of an electronic record.

Certified Copy means a copy of original information that has been verified, as indicated by dated signature, as an exact copy having all of the same attributes and information as the original.

Commit means a saving action, which creates or modifies, or an action which deletes, an electronic record or portion of an electronic record. An example is pressing the key of a keyboard that causes information to be saved to durable medium.

Computerized System means, for the purpose of this guidance, computer hardware, software, and associated documents (e.g., user manual) that create, modify, maintain, archive, retrieve, or transmit in digital form information related to the conduct of a clinical trial.

Direct Entry means recording data where an electronic record is the original capture of the data. Examples are the keying by an individual of original observations into the system, or automatic recording by the system of the output of a balance that measures subject's body weight.

Electronic Case Report Form (e-CRF) means an auditable electronic record designed to record information required by the clinical trial protocol to be reported to the sponsor on each trial subject.

Electronic Patient Diary means an electronic record into which a subject participating in a clinical trial directly enters observations or directly responds to an evaluation checklist.

Electronic Record means any combination of text, graphics, data, audio, pictorial, or any other information representation in digital form that is created, modified, maintained, archived, retrieved, or distributed by a computer system.

Electronic Signature means a computer data compilation of any symbol or series of symbols, executed, adopted, or authorized by an individual to be the legally binding equivalent of the individual's handwritten signature.

Software Validation means confirmation by examination and provision of objective evidence that software specifications conform to user needs and intended uses, and that the particular requirements implemented through the software can be consistently fulfilled. For the purposes of this document, design level validation is that portion of the software validation that takes place in parts of the software life cycle before the software is delivered to the end user.

Source Documents means original documents and records including, but not limited to, hospital records, clinical and office charts, laboratory notes, memoranda, subjects' diaries or evaluation checklists, pharmacy dispensing records, recorded data from automated instruments, copies or transcriptions certified after verification as being accurate and complete, microfiches, photographic negatives, microfilm or magnetic media, x-rays, subject files, and records kept at the pharmacy, at the laboratories, and at medico-technical departments involved in the clinical trial.

Transmit means, for the purposes of this guidance, to transfer data within or among clinical study sites, contract research organizations, data management centers, or sponsors. Other Agency guidance covers transmission from sponsors to the Agency.

III. General Principles

A. Each study protocol should identify at which steps a computerized system will be used to create, modify, maintain, archive, retrieve, or transmit data.

B. For each study, documentation should identify what software and, if known, what hardware is to be used in computerized systems that create, modify, maintain, archive, retrieve, or transmit data. This documentation should be retained as part of study records.

C. Source documents should be retained to enable a reconstruction and evaluation of the trial.

D. When original observations are entered directly into a computerized system, the electronic record is the source document.

E. The design of a computerized system should ensure that all applicable regulatory requirements for recordkeeping and record retention in clinical trials are met with the same degree of confidence as is provided with paper systems.

F. Clinical investigators should retain either the original or a certified copy of all source documents sent to a sponsor or contract research organization, including query resolution correspondence.

G. Any change to a record required to be maintained should not obscure the original information. The record should clearly indicate that a change was made and clearly provide a means to locate and read the prior information.

H. Changes to data that are stored on electronic media will always require an audit trail, in accordance with 21 CFR 11.10(e). Documentation should include who made the changes, when, and why they were made.

I. The FDA may inspect all records that are intended to support submissions to the Agency, regardless of how they were created or maintained.

J. Data should be retrievable in such a fashion that all information regarding each individual subject in a study is attributable to that subject.

K. Computerized systems should be designed: (1) So that all requirements assigned to these systems in a study protocol are satisfied (e.g., data are recorded in metric units, requirements that the study be blinded); and,

(2) to preclude errors in data creation, modification, maintenance, archiving, retrieval, or transmission.

Security measures should be in place to prevent unauthorized access to the data and to the computerized system.

IV. Standard Operating Procedures

Standard Operating Procedures (SOPs) pertinent to the use of the computerized system should be available on site.

SOPs should be established for, but not limited to:

- System Setup/Installation
- Data Collection and Handling
- System Maintenance
- Data Backup, Recovery, and Contingency Plans
- Security
- Change Control

Data Entry

A. Electronic Signatures

1. To ensure that individuals have the authority to proceed with data entry, the data entry system should be designed so that individuals need to enter electronic signatures, such as combined identification codes/passwords or biometric-based electronic signatures, at the start of a data entry session.

2. The data entry system should also be designed to ensure attributability. Therefore, each entry to an electronic record, including any change, should be made under the electronic signature of the individual making that entry. However, this does not necessarily mean a separate electronic signature for each entry or change. For example, a single electronic signature may cover multiple entries or changes.

a. The printed name of the individual who enters data should be displayed by the data entry screen throughout the data entry session. This is intended to preclude the possibility of a different individual inadvertently entering data under someone else=s name.

   If the name displayed by the screen during a data entry session is not that of the person entering the data, then that individual should log on under his or her own name before continuing.

3. Individuals should only work under their own passwords or other access keys and should not share these with others. Individuals should not log on to the system in order to provide another person access to the system.

4. Passwords or other access keys should be changed at established intervals.

5. When someone leaves a workstation, the person should log off the system. Failing this, an automatic log off may be appropriate for long idle periods. For short periods of inactivity, there should be some kind of automatic protection against unauthorized data entry. An example could be an automatic screen saver that prevents data entry until a password is entered.

B. Audit Trails

1. Section 21 CFR 11.10(e) requires persons who use electronic record systems to maintain an audit trail as one of the procedures to protect the authenticity, integrity, and, when appropriate, the confidentiality of electronic records.

a. Persons must use secure, computer-generated, time-stamped audit trails to independently record the date and time of operator entries and actions that create, modify, or delete electronic records. A record is created when it is saved to durable media, as described under "commit" in Section II, Definitions.

b. Audit trails must be retained for a period at least as long as that required for the subject electronic records (e.g., the study data and records to which they pertain) and must be available for agency review and copying.

2. Personnel who create, modify, or delete electronic records should not be able to modify the audit trails.

3. Clinical investigators should retain either the original or a certified copy of audit trails.

4. FDA personnel should be able to read audit trails both at the study site and at any other location where associated electronic study records are maintained.

5. Audit trails should be created incrementally, in chronological order, and in a manner that does not allow new audit trail information to overwrite existing data in violation of §11.10(e).

C. Date/Time Stamps

Controls should be in place to ensure that the system's date and time are correct.

The ability to change the date or time should be limited to authorized personnel and such personnel should be notified if a system date or time discrepancy is detected. Changes to date or time should be documented.

Dates and times are to be local to the activity being documented and should include the year, month, day, hour, and minute. The Agency encourages establishments to synchronize systems to the date and time provided by trusted third parties.

Clinical study computerized systems will likely be used in multi-center trials, perhaps located in different time zones. Calculation of the local time stamp may be derived in such cases from a remote server located in a different time zone.

VI. System Features

A. Systems used for direct entry of data should include features that will facilitate the collection of quality data.

Prompts, flags, or other help features within the computerized system should be used to encourage consistent use of clinical terminology and to alert the user to data that are out of acceptable range. Features that automatically enter data into a field when that field is bypassed should not be used.

Electronic patient diaries and e-CRFs should be designed to allow users to make annotations. Annotations add to data quality by allowing ad hoc information to be captured. This information may be valuable in the event of an adverse reaction or unexpected result. The record should clearly indicate who recorded the annotations and when (date and time).

B. Systems used for direct entry of data should be designed to include features that will facilitate the inspection and review of data. Data tags (e.g., different color, different font, flags) should be used to indicate which data have been changed or deleted, as documented in the audit trail.

C. Retrieval of Data

Recognizing that computer products may be discontinued or supplanted by newer (possibly incompatible) systems, it is nonetheless vital that sponsors retain the ability to retrieve and review the data recorded by the older systems. This may be achieved by maintaining support for the older systems or transcribing data to the newer systems.

When migrating to newer systems, it is important to generate accurate and complete copies of study data and collateral information relevant to data integrity. This information would include, for example, audit trails and computational methods used to derive the data. Any data retrieval software, script, or query logic used for the purpose of manipulating, querying, or extracting data for report generating purposes should be documented and maintained for the life of the report. The transcription process needs to be validated.

D. Reconstruction of Study

FDA expects to be able to reconstruct a study. This applies not only to the data, but also how the data were obtained or managed. Therefore, all versions of application software, operating systems, and software development tools involved in processing of data or records should be available as long as data or records associated with these versions are required to be retained. Sponsors may retain these themselves or may contract for the vendors to retain the ability to run (but not necessarily support) the software. Although FDA expects sponsors or vendors to retain the ability to run older versions of software, the agency acknowledges that, in some cases, it will be difficult for sponsors and vendors to run older computerized systems.

VII. Security

A. Physical Security

In addition to internal safeguards built into the system, external safeguards should be in place to ensure that access to the computerized system and to the data is restricted to authorized personnel.

Staff should be thoroughly aware of system security measures and the importance of limiting access to authorized personnel.

SOPs should be in place for handling and storing the system to prevent unauthorized access.

B. Logical Security

Access to the data at the clinical site should be restricted and monitored through the system's software with its required log-on, security procedures, and audit trail. The data should not be altered, browsed, queried, or reported via external software applications that do not enter through the protective system software.

There should be a cumulative record that indicates, for any point in time, the names of authorized personnel, their titles, and a description of their access privileges. The record should be in the study documentation accessible at the site.

If a sponsor supplies computerized systems exclusively for clinical trials, the systems should remain dedicated to the purpose for which they were intended and validated.

If a computerized system being used for the clinical study is part of a system normally used for other purposes, efforts should be made to ensure that the study software is logically and physically isolated as necessary to preclude unintended interaction with non-study software. If any of the software programs are changed the system should be evaluated to determine the effect of the changes on logical security.

Controls should be in place to prevent, detect, and mitigate effects of computer viruses on study data and software.

System Dependability

The sponsor should ensure and document that computerized systems conform to the sponsor's established requirements for completeness, accuracy, reliability, and consistent intended performance.

A. Systems documentation should be readily available at the site where clinical trials are conducted. Such documentation should provide an overall description of computerized systems and the relationship of hardware, software, and physical environment.

B. FDA may inspect documentation, possessed by a regulated company, that demonstrates validation of software. The study sponsor is responsible, if requested, for making such documentation available at the time of inspection at the site where software is used. Clinical investigators are not generally responsible for validation unless they originated or modified software.

1. For software purchased off-the-shelf, most of the validation should have been done by the company that wrote the software. The sponsor or contract research organization should have documentation (either original validation documents or on-site vendor audit documents) of this design level validation by the vendor, and should have itself performed functional testing (e.g., by use of test data sets) and researched known software limitations, problems, and defect corrections.

In the special case of database and spreadsheet software that is (1) purchased off-the-shelf, (2) designed for and widely used for general purposes, (3) unmodified, and (4) not being used for direct entry of data, the sponsor or contract research organization may not have documentation of design level validation. However, the sponsor or contract research organization should have itself performed functional testing (e.g., by use of test data sets) and researched known software limitations, problems, and defect corrections.

2. Documentation important to demonstrate software validation includes:

- Written design specification that describes what the software is intended to do and how it is intended to do it;

- A written test plan based on the design specification, including both structural and functional analysis; and,

- Test results and an evaluation of how these results demonstrate that the predetermined design specification has been met.

C. Change Control

Written procedures should be in place to ensure that changes to the computerized system such as software upgrades, equipment or component replacement, or new instrumentation will maintain the integrity of the data or the integrity of protocols.

The impact of any change to the system should be evaluated and a decision made regarding the need to revalidate. Revalidation should be performed for changes that exceed operational limits or design specifications.

All changes to the system should be documented.

IX. System Controls

A. Software Version Control

Measures should be in place to ensure that versions of software used to generate, collect, maintain, and transmit data are the versions that are stated in the systems documentation.

B. Contingency Plans

Written procedures should describe contingency plans for continuing the study by alternate means in the event of failure of the computerized system.

C. Backup and Recovery of Electronic Records

Backup and recovery procedures should be clearly outlined in the SOPs and be sufficient to protect against data loss. Records should be backed up regularly in a way that would prevent a catastrophic loss and ensure the quality and integrity of the data.

Backup records should be stored at a secure location specified in the SOPs. Storage is typically offsite or in a building separate from the original records.

Backup and recovery logs should be maintained to facilitate an assessment of the nature and scope of data loss resulting from a system failure.

X. Training of Personnel

A. Qualifications

Each person who enters or processes data should have the education, training, and experience or any combination thereof necessary to perform the assigned functions.

Individuals responsible for monitoring the trial should have education, training, and experience in the use of the computerized system necessary to adequately monitor the trial.

B. Training

Training should be provided to individuals in the specific operations that they are to perform.

Training should be conducted by qualified individuals on a continuing basis, as needed, to ensure familiarity with the computerized system and with any changes to the system during the course of the study.

C. Documentation

Employee education, training, and experience should be documented.

XI. Records Inspection

A. FDA may inspect all records that are intended to support submissions to the Agency, regardless of how they were created or maintained. Therefore, systems should be able to generate accurate and complete copies of records in both human readable and electronic form suitable for inspection, review, and copying by the Agency. Persons should contact the Agency if there is any doubt about what file formats and media the Agency can read and copy.

B. The sponsor should be able to provide hardware and software as necessary for FDA personnel to inspect the electronic documents and audit trail at the site where an FDA inspection is taking place.

XII. Certification of Electronic Signatures

As required by 21 CFR 11.100(c), persons using electronic signatures to meet an FDA signature requirement shall, prior to or at the time of such use, certify to the agency that the electronic signatures in their system, used on or after August 20, 1997, are intended to be the legally binding equivalent of traditional handwritten signatures.

As set forth in 21 CFR 11.100(c), the certification shall be submitted in paper form signed with a traditional handwritten signature to the Office of Regional Operations (HFC-100), 5600 Fishers Lane, Rockville Maryland 20857. The certification is to be submitted prior to or at the time electronic signatures are used. However, a single certification may cover all electronic signatures used by persons in a given organization. This certification is a legal document created by persons to acknowledge that their electronic signatures have the same legal significance as their traditional handwritten signatures. An acceptable certification may take the following form:

"Pursuant to Section 11.100 of Title 21 of the Code of Federal Regulations, this is to certify that [name of organization] intends that all electronic signatures executed by our employees, agents, or representatives, located anywhere in the world, are the legally binding equivalent of traditional handwritten signatures."

XIII. References

FDA, Software Development Activities, 1987.

FDA, Guideline for the Monitoring of Clinical Investigations, 1988.

FDA, Guidance for Industry: Good Target Animal Practices: Clinical Investigators and Monitors, 1997.

FDA, Compliance Program Guidance Manual, "Compliance Program 7348.810 - Sponsors, Contract Research Organizations and Monitors," October 30, 1998.

FDA, Compliance Program Guidance Manual, "Compliance Program 7348.811 - Bioresearch Monitoring - Clinical Investigators," September 2, 1998.

FDA, Information Sheets for Institutional Review Boards and Clinical Investigators, 1998.

FDA, Glossary of Computerized System and Software Development Terminology, 1995.

FDA, 21 CFR Part 11, Electronic Records; Electronic Signatures; Final Rule. Federal Register Vol. 62, No. 54, 13429, March 20, 1997.

FDA, [draft] Guidance for Industry: General Principles of Software Validation, draft 1997.

International Conference on Harmonisation, Good Clinical Practice: Consolidated Guideline, Federal Register Vol 62, No. 90, 25711, May 9, 1997.

ABOUT CENTERWATCH

CenterWatch is a Boston-based publishing and information services company that focuses on the clinical trials industry. We provide a variety of information services used by pharmaceutical and biotechnology companies, CROs, SMOs and investigative sites involved in the management and conduct of clinical trials. CenterWatch also provides educational materials for clinical research professionals, health professionals and for health consumers. We provide market research and market intelligence services that many major companies have retained to help develop new business strategies, to guide the implementation of new clinical research-related initiatives and to assist in due diligence activities. Some of our top publications and services are described below. For a comprehensive listing with detailed information about our publications and services, please visit our web site at www.centerwatch.com. You can also contact us at (800) 765-9647 for subscription and order information.

22 Thomson Place · Boston, MA 02210
Phone (617) 856-5900 · Fax (617) 856-5901
www.centerwatch.com

CenterWatch Training Manuals and Directories

The Investigator's Guide to Clinical Research, 3rd edition
This 250-page step-by-step manual is filled with tips, instructions and insights for health professionals interested in conducting clinical trials. The *Investigator's Guide* is designed to help the novice clinical investigator get involved in conducting clinical trials. The guide is also a valuable resource for experienced investigative sites looking for ways to improve and increase their involvement and success in clinical research. Developed in accordance with ACCME, readers can apply for CME credits. An exam is provided online.

How to Find & Secure Clinical Grants
This 28-page guidebook is an ideal resource for healthcare professionals interested in conducting clinical trials. The guidebook provides tips and insights for new and experienced investigative sites to compete more effectively for clinical study grants.

How to Grow Your Investigative Site: A Guide to Operating and Expanding a Successful Clinical Research Center
This 300-page book is an ideal resource for clinical investigators interested in expanding their clinical trials operations in order to establish a more successful and effective research enterprise. Written by Barry Miskin, M.D., and Ann Neuer, the book is filled with practical case examples, insights, tips and reference resources designed to assist investigators and study personnel in growing a viable and successful clinical research business. Readers can apply for CME credits. An exam is provided online.

A Guide to Patient Recruitment:
Today's Best Practices and Proven Strategies
This 350-page manual is designed to help clinical research professionals improve the effectiveness of their patient recruitment efforts. Written by Diana Anderson, Ph.D., with contributions from 15 industry experts and thought leaders, this guide offers real world, practical recruitment strategies and tactics. It is considered an invaluable resource for educating professionals who manage and conduct clinical research about ways to plan and execute effective patient recruitment and retention efforts. Readers can apply for CME credits. An exam is provided online.

Protecting Study Volunteers in Research, 2nd edition
A Manual For Investigative Sites
The second edition of our top-selling manual has doubled in size to address current and emerging issues that are critical to our system of human subject protection oversight. *Protecting Study Volunteers in Research* is a suggested educational resource by NIH and FDA (source: NIH Notice OD-00-039, 2000, page 37841; Federal Registry 2002) and is designed to help organizations provide the highest standards of safe and ethical treatment of study volun-

teers. Written specifically for academic institutions and IRBs actively involved in clinical trials, the manual is also applicable to independent investigative sites. The book has been developed in accordance with the ACCME. Readers can apply for CME credits or Nursing Credit Hours. An exam is provided with each manual and is also available online.

Ensuring a HIPAA-Compliant Informed Consent Process

Both an instruction manual and a reference resource, this 158-page book provides detailed guidelines on how to manage and conduct a HIPAA-compliant and IRB-acceptable informed consent process. The guide includes sample language and templates for the HIPAA Authorization Form and informed consent forms for use in a variety of clinical research studies including genetic testing, tissue banking and assent. An extensive glossary of terms for use in preparing informed consent documents and convenient and easy-to-reference regulatory guidelines are also included.

The CRA's Guide to Monitoring Clinical Research

This 450+ page CE-accredited book is an ideal resource for novice and experienced CRAs, as well as professionals interested in pursuing a career as study monitors. The CRA's Guide covers important topics along with updated regulations, guidelines and worksheets, including resources such as: 21 CFR Parts 50, 54, 56 & 312 Guidelines, various checklists (monitoring visit, site evaluation, informed consent) and a study documentation file verification log. This manual will be routinely referenced throughout the CRA's career.

The New CenterWatch Drugs in Clinical Trials Database

The *Drugs in Clinical Trials Database* is a comprehensive web-based, searchable resource offering detailed profiles of new investigational treatments in phase I through III clinical trials. Updated daily, this online and searchable directory provides information on more than 2,000 drugs for more than 600 indications worldwide in a well-organized and easy-to-reference format. Detailed profile information is provided for each drug. A separate section is provided on pediatric treatments. The *Drugs in Clinical Trials Database* is an ideal online resource for industry professionals to use for monitoring the performance of drugs in clinical trials; tracking competitors' development activity; identifying development partners; and identifying clinical study grant opportunities.

The 2003 CenterWatch Directory of the Clinical Trials Industry

This comprehensive directory holds more than 1,000 pages of contact information and detailed company profiles for a wide range of organizations and individuals involved in the clinical trials industry. It is considered the authoritative reference resource for organizations involved in designing, managing, conducting and supporting clinical trials.

Profiles of Service Providers on the
CenterWatch Clinical Trials Listing Service™
The CenterWatch web site (www.centerwatch.com) attracts tens of thousands of sponsor and CRO company representatives every month that are looking for experienced service providers and investigative sites to manage and conduct their clinical trials. No registration is required. Sponsors and CROs use this online directory free of charge. The CenterWatch web site offers all contract service providers—both CROs and investigative sites—the opportunity to present more information than any other Internet-based service available. This service is an ideal way to secure new contracts and clinical study grants.

An Industry in Evolution
This 250-page sourcebook provides extensive data and facts documenting clinical trial industry trends and benchmarked practices. The material—charts, statistics and analytical reports—is presented in an easy-to-reference format. This important and valuable resource is used for developing business strategies and plans, for preparing presentations and for conducting business and market intelligence.

CenterWatch Compilation Reports Series
These topic specific reports provide comprehensive, in-depth features, original research and analyses and fact-based company/institution business and financial profiles. Reports are available on Site Management Organizations, Academic Medical Centers, and Contract Research Organizations. Spanning nearly five years of in-depth coverage and analyses, these reports provide valuable insights into company strategies, market dynamics and successful business practices. Ideal for business planning and for market intelligence/market research activities.

The CenterWatch Patient Education Series

As part of ongoing reforms in human subject protection oversight, institutional and independent IRBs and research centers are actively identifying educational programs and assessment mechanisms to use with their study volunteers. These initiatives are of particular interest among those IRBs that are applying for voluntary accreditation with the Association for the Accreditation of Human Research Protection Programs (AAHRPP) and the National Committee for Quality Assurance (NCQA). CenterWatch offers a variety of educational communications for use by IRB and clinical research professionals.

Informed Consent™: A Guide to the Risks and Benefits of Volunteering for Clinical Trials

This comprehensive 300-page reference resource is designed to assist patients and health consumers in understanding the clinical trial process and their rights and recourse as study volunteers. Based on extensive review and input from bioethicists, regulatory and industry experts, the guide provides facts, insights and case examples designed to assist individuals in making informed decisions about participating in clinical trials. The guide is an ideal educational reference that research and IRB professionals can use to review with their study volunteers, to address volunteer questions and concerns, and to further build relationships with the patient community. Professionals also refer to this guide for assistance in responding to the media.

Volunteering For a Clinical Trial

This easy-to-read, six-page patient education brochure is designed for research centers to provide consistent, professional and unbiased educational information for their potential clinical study subjects. The brochure is IRB approved and is used by sponsors, CROs and investigative sites to help set patient expectations about participating in clinical trials. *Volunteering for a Clinical Trial* can be distributed in a variety of ways including direct mailings to patients, displays in waiting rooms, or as handouts to guide discussions. The brochure can be customized with company logos and custom information.

A Word from Study Volunteers: Opinions and Experiences of Clinical Trial Participants

This straightforward and easy-to-read ten-page pamphlet reviews the results of a survey conducted among more than 1,200 clinical research volunteers. This brochure presents first-hand experiences from clinical trial volunteers. It offers valuable insights for individuals interested in participating in a clinical trial. The brochure can be customized with company logos and custom information.

The CenterWatch Clinical Trials Listing Service™

Now in its seventh year of operation, *The CenterWatch Clinical Trials Listing Service™* provides the largest and most comprehensive listing of Industry- and Government-sponsored clinical trials on the Internet. In 2002, the CenterWatch web site—along with numerous coordinated online and print affiliations—is expected to reach more than 8 million Americans. *The CenterWatch Clinical Trials Listing Service™* provides an international listing of more than 42,000, ongoing and IRB-approved phase I–IV clinical trials.

CenterWatch Periodicals

CenterWatch

Our award-winning monthly newsletter provides pharmaceutical and biotechnology companies, CROs, SMOs, academic institutions, research centers and the investment community with in-depth business news and insights, feature articles on trends and clinical research practices, original market intelligence and analysis, as well as grant lead information for investigative sites.

CWWeekly

This weekly newsletter, available as a fax or in electronic format, reports on the top stories and breaking news in the clinical trials industry. Each week the newsletter includes business headlines, financial information, market intelligence, drug pipeline and clinical trial results.

JobWatch

This web-based resource at www.centerwatch.com, complemented by a print publication, provides comprehensive listings of career and educational opportunities in the clinical trials industry, including a searchable resume database service and online CE- and CME-accredited learning modules. Companies use *JobWatch* regularly to identify qualified clinical research professionals and career and educational services.

CenterWatch Intelligence Services

Market Intelligence Reports and Services

With nearly a decade of experience gathering original data and writing about all aspects of the clinical research enterprise, the *CenterWatch Market Intelligence Department* is uniquely positioned to provide a wide range of market research services designed to assist organizations in making more informed strategic business decisions that impact their clinical research activities. Our clients include major biopharmaceutical companies, CROs and contract service providers, site networks, investment analysts and management consulting firms. CenterWatch brings unprecedented industry knowledge, extensive industry-wide relationships and expertise gathering, analyzing and presenting primary and secondary quantitative and qualitative data. Along with our custom research projects for clients, CenterWatch also facilitates on-site management forums designed to explore critical business trends and their implications. These sessions offer a wealth of data and a unique opportunity for senior professionals to think about business problems in new ways.

TrialWatch Site-Identification Service

Several hundred sponsor and CRO companies use the TrialWatch service to identify prospective investigative sites to conduct their upcoming clinical trials. Every month, companies post bulletins of their phase I–IV development programs that are actively seeking clinical investigators. These bulletins are included in *CenterWatch*—our flagship monthly publication that reaches as many as 25,000 experienced investigators every month. Use of the *TrialWatch* service is FREE.

Content License Services

CenterWatch offers both database content and static text under license. All CenterWatch content can be seamlessly integrated into your company Internet, Intranet or Extranet web site(s) with or without frames. Our database offerings include: the *Clinical Trials Listing Service™, Clinical Trial Results, Drugs in Clinical Trials, Newly Approved Drugs, The Clinical Trial Industry Directory,* and *CW-Mobile* for Wireless OS® Devices. Our static text offerings include: an editorial feature on background information on clinical trials and a glossary of clinical trial terminology.

ABOUT THE AUTHORS

Rebecca Daniels Kush, Ph.D. is a founder and the current president of the Clinical Data Interchange Standards Consortium (CDISC), a non-profit organization dedicated to the development of global data interchange standards to support the acquisition, exchange, submission and archive of clinical trial data.

Dr. Kush earned a Ph.D. in Physiology and Pharmacology from the University of California (UCSD) School of Medicine in La Jolla, CA. She conducted basic clinical research as a Fellow at the NIH facility in Phoenix, Ariz. and later for Baxter-Travenol in Japan. In addition, she worked for the Product Planning Department for Eisai, Co. in Tokyo and later as a consultant for this pharmaceutical company while in France and the U.S.

Dr. Kush has more than 25 years of experience in clinical research and activities related to drug development. After her employment abroad, she worked at Pharmaco, an international contract research organization. Her latest positions at Pharmaco were coordinator of its corporate process analysis and redesign effort and director, clinical processes and standards.

Prior to dedicating full-time as president of CDISC, Dr. Kush founded a consulting company, Catalysis, Inc. Focus areas for her consulting are strategy, process analysis and redesign, particularly associated with electronic clinical trials; project management infrastructure and training; implementation of enabling technologies; and clinical trial metrics.

Through the formal relationship between CDISC and Health Level 7 (HL7), Dr. Kush is a member of HL7. She is also a member of DIA, SCDM, and ACRP. She has served on the Steering Committee of North America for

DIA for three years and has chaired the program development for numerous workshops in the areas of EDC, eClinical Trials, and Data Standards.

Paul A. Bleicher, M.D., Ph.D., is chairman and founder of Phase Forward Incorporated, a clinical trial data management software company.

Dr. Bleicher earned his M.D. and Ph.D. from the University of Rochester and trained in internal medicine and dermatology at Harvard Medical School. He completed a post-doctoral fellowship in molecular immunology at the Dana Farber Cancer Institute and was subsequently appointed an assistant professor of dermatology at Massachusetts General Hospital and Harvard Medical School. He is a board certified dermatologist.

Prior to founding Phase Forward, he worked at Parexel International, as a medical monitor and as director, early phase services. Later, he served as vice president of clinical affairs for Alpha-Beta Technology, where he guided the clinical development and testing of novel carbohydrate-based immunotherapeutic compounds.

Dr. Bleicher currently serves as chair of the DIA Steering Committee of North America and serves as an *ex officio* member of the Board of Directors. Dr. Bleicher serves on the editorial boards of the *Drug Information Journal* and *Applied Clinical Trials*, for which he also writes a regular technology column. He is a member of the Dean's Advisory Council for the School of Science of Rensselaer Polytechnic Institute.

Wayne R. Kubick is technical director and an original member of the Board of Directors for CDISC who has led the activities of two CDISC data modeling teams. In his spare time he serves as a vice president, consulting with Lincoln Technologies of Boston, Mass., specializing in clinical data architectures, data mining, electronic regulatory submissions, electronic data capture and information technology strategies and processes for clinical development. He was formerly CIO and vice president of information technology at Parexel International where he introduced new technologies for clinical research including RDE, Image Recognition, CANDAs, and IVR systems. He has also worked for BBN Software Products and The Analytical Sciences Corporation. Mr. Kubick possesses nearly 20 years of information systems experience and holds a B.A. from the University of Illinois and an MBA from Boston University.

Stephen T. Kush has more than 25 years of experience in technology, engineering and manufacturing. He has worked for Texas Instruments, Sperry Flight Systems and Schlumberger in a variety of research and product development areas including fiber optics, communications and real time acquisition systems. This experience included work assignments in Japan and France that provided a more global perspective. In addition to specific product development activities, Mr. Kush has managed quality assurance, information services and technology departments that supported the product development process. For the past 10 years, Mr. Kush has focused on optimizing the processes required to bring innovative products to the market-place and has served as a consultant for companies in the healthcare indus-try. He received a B.S. and M.S. in electrical engineering from the University of Texas at Austin and undertook additional graduate study at the University of Arizona Optical Sciences Department.

Ronald Marks, Ph.D., is professor of biostatistics at the University of Florida and president of MarCon Global Data Solutions. He received his MS and Ph.D. in Statistics from the University of Florida. He has been involved in clinical research throughout his academic career and has collaborated on the development of a web-based clinical research system since 1996. He has been co-principal investigator on a 22,000-patient phase IV clinical trial in 10 countries conducted by the University of Florida using this technology. Also, for the past two years has been involved in the commercialization of the technology.

Stephen A. Raymond, Ph.D., is the chief scientific officer, quality officer and founder of PHT Corporation in Charlestown, Mass. Dr. Raymond received a BS degree in physiology from Stanford University and a Ph.D. in neuro-physiology from MIT in 1969. He held faculty appointments in electrical engineering and computer science at MIT from 1970 to 2001, where he taught courses in analog circuit design, systems and neuroscience. Since 1981 Dr. Raymond has been an assistant professor of anesthesia doing research at Harvard Medical School and was a neurophysiologist at Brigham and Women's Hospital until 2002. He has invented various electronic and mechanical instruments, and holds several patents.

He joined Personal Health Technologies Corporation (PHT) as chief sci-entific officer in June of 1997. At PHT he has been developing techniques for longitudinal monitoring of patients in clinical research. He believes that mobile data capture appliances with enhanced features for capturing elec-tronic source will transform clinical trials, enabling more and better scien-tific research on human subjects to be accomplished. In recent articles and conference presentations he has considered the regulatory and privacy objectives of clinical trials and how data integrity can be ensured for elec-tronic source technologies.

Barbara Tardiff, M.D., is vice president, clinical informatics at Regeneron Pharmaceuticals, a biopharmaceutical company. Dr. Tardiff received her medical and graduate science education at Yale University and an MBA at Duke University. She is board certified in pediatrics and anesthesiology with subspecialty training in cardiothoracic anesthesia. She completed a clinical research fellowship at the Duke Clinical Research Institute. Prior to joining Regeneron, she was vice president, biomedical informatics, at iBiomatics, a subsidiary of SAS Institute and chief strategist for the biopharmaceutical industry at SAS. Dr. Tardiff was previously the director of clinical data integration at the Duke Clinical Research Institute. She remains a member of the DCRI faculty and an assistant consulting professor at Duke University.

Dr. Tardiff is also active in establishing standards through CDISC, the Clinical Data Interchange Standards Consortium, and HL7 (Health Level 7). She is co-chair and a member of the HL7 Regulated Clinical Research Information Management (RCRIM) Technical Committee. She is an expert in integration, deployment and evaluation of biomedical data and has participated in a broad range of clinical care and scientific and operational clinical research study activities.

NOTES

NOTES

NOTES

NOTES

NOTES

NOTES

NOTES

NOTES

NOTES

NOTES

NOTES

NOTES

NOTES

NOTES